SEVEN AMAZING CUTTING-EDGE THERAPIES

By
Michael Watts

Illustrated by
Gray Jolliffe

First Printing: April 2017

ISBN-13 978-1545079898

Disclaimer

The author and publisher cannot be held responsible for any actions taken by the reader as a result of any reliance on the text, which is taken entirely at the reader's own risk. Readers are advised to consult medical practitioners for any physical or psychological condition that may require medical attention.

The author and publisher disclaim all responsibility for any problems that may arise from any therapies described here, whether during unsupervised, self-treatment or when visiting an appropriate, qualified medical practitioner. This book is intended for entertainment and information and should not be used for diagnosis or treatment. The author is not a medical doctor.

GRAY JOLLIFFE

Currently, his work includes Chloe & Co in the Daily Mail

Among the numerous authors whose books Gray has illustrated are the following:

1. Sir Terry Pratchett. Worldwide sales of his books, translated into 37 languages, now stand at 70 million.

2. Charles Roger Hargreaves: Gray illustrated around ten books for Hargreaves, who is best remembered for the *Mr. Men & Little Miss series*. Translated into 20 languages, Hargreaves is Britain's third best-selling author of all time having sold more than 100 million books.

3. Bruce Fogle World's best-selling practicing vet with books in over 35 languages.

4. Cathy Hopkins: Collaborated with Gray Jolliffe on a series of humour books. 55 books published in 33 different countries.

5. Peter Mayle: Gray illustrated several books for Peter. (British Book Awards named *A Year in Provence* Best Travel Book of the Year).

6. Celia Haddon: British journalist and author. Her 40 published books include a series of best-selling books about cats, most successful of which is *One Hundred Ways for a Cat to Train its Human*.

MICHAEL WATTS

Michael Watts graduated with honors in 1980 with a BSc in Experimental Psychology, (Sussex University). An independent scholar and writer, he has researched widely in philosophy, his specialist interest being in the affinity between East Asian non-dualist philosophy and Existentialism and the implications this has for everyday existence. Over the years, he has also maintained a passionate interest in Qigong and Tai Chi and is a certified instructor of both disciplines. Hobbies: Hanggliding

Michael has contributed articles to various magazines and national newspapers in the UK, USA, Canada, Australia and Sweden; these have included USA Today, Fitness Magazine, Toronto Sun, The Sunday Times Magazine, Sunday Telegraph, Daily Mirror and Bella. And in Australia: New Idea, Cosmopolitan and Womans Day.

His numerous television appearances include ITV, BBC 1 and Sky News and he has also been a frequent BBC radio guest.

His publications have been very well received by his peers in the academic community worldwide.

Book Publications since Year 2000:

1. The Philosophy of Heidegger, (Continental European Philosophy Series) by Michael Watts, Acumen Publishing, April 2011. (Also published as an e book, September 2014, under same title).

2. Kierkegaard (Philosophers), by Michael Watts, Oneworld Publications, Oxford 2003. (Also published as an e book, September 2014, title: Kierkegaard: An Essential Introduction).

3. Heidegger: A Beginner's Guide, by Michael Watts, Hodder and Stoughton Educational, London, 2001. (Also published as an e book, November 2014, title: Heidegger: An Essential Guide for Beginners)

4. Heidegger: A Beginner's Guide, Spanish Language Edition: Heidegger Guia para Jovenes, (Michael Watts) Logues Ediciones, Madrid, 2003)

5. Heidegger: A Beginner's Guide, Korean Language Edition (Michael Watts): Korean Translation copyright by Random House Joong-Ang Inc. Seoul, 2006.

CONTENTS

Gray Jolliffe 5

Michael Watts 7

Foreword 11

Introduction 13

Chapter One: Professor Nutt & Psychedelic Therapy 19

Chapter Two: Dr Berceli's Trauma Therapy 83

Chapter Three: Canine Diagnostics 97

Chapter Four: Epley Omniax Vertigo Therapy 107

Chapter Five: Helminth Therapy 121

Chapter Six: Cutting Edge Apitherapy 145

Chapter Seven: Beer-Spa Therapy 157

FOREWORD

Interesting, intriguing and entertaining! An exposé of cutting-edge medical treatments. Dogs diagnosing earliest stage cancer; Psychedelic therapy that can successfully dissolve destructive thought patterns and relieve treatment-resistant depression; an innovative approach inspired by observations of animal behaviour in the wild, that can effectively treat seemingly intractable PTSD. A recommended read both for professionals and also for the general reader.

One should always reconsider old truths and habits, and in a scientific manner examine them.

Dr Joakim Litzberg M.D. (Sweden)

Michael's attempt to articulate a concise summary of the TRE process is quite admirable. He maintains a factually accurate description of TRE, covering the most salient components of this physical approach to relieving stress, tension and trauma symptoms, while including the theoretical and practical foundations upon which TRE is based.

Dr David Berceli

INTRODUCTION

Conventional doctors today are, for a variety of reasons, often hesitant in recommending treatments within the area of "Complimentary Alternative Medicine". This is because it is normally not included in their training, so they have not experienced or researched its potential. And their caution is sometimes justified, because although solid empirically-based evidence exists for some CAM therapies, such as acupuncture, which is already on offer by the NHS; many of these treatments are still poorly understood or simply cannot yet be comprehended from a scientific point of view. This means that key questions about them remain unanswered.

More importantly, overenthusiastic CAM practitioners are frequently prone towards making exaggerated claims about the efficacy of their treatments, without being able to offer solid data to back them up. What makes things worse is that some even insist that you forgo conventional treatments entirely, which in some cases can – and sometimes does – have potentially lethal consequences.

Indeed, the word "complimentary" intrinsically points out that these are treatments that should be considered only in conjunction with, and not to the exclusion of conventional medical approaches.

Sometimes, the apparent efficacy of a CAM treatment is due merely to the patient's faith, or to the fact that certain medical problems are cyclical. For example, certain allergies and illnesses such as multiple sclerosis, arthritis and gastrointestinal problems, like irritable bowel syndrome, all have their ups and downs. If a sufferer seeks a particular CAM treatment just when the 'down phase' of a cycle is ending, and the up phase is commencing, then they are likely to attribute their improvements to a therapy which might in fact have no useful medical benefits whatsoever. This tends not to occur in conventional treatments which are rooted in controlled trials that exclude the 'cyclical effect' of illnesses.

Additionally, many diseases are self-limiting. For instance some types of cold virus only last around six or seven days, and if a person is ignorant of this fact, and always uses a particular 'alternative' cure whenever they catch a cold, then they might believe that they owe their recovery each time to the 'medicine', when in fact their improvement may have been merely due to the passage of time.

Readers should always keep in mind that the 'Placebo Effect' can contribute significantly to a person's recovery , independent of the intrinsic effects of the particular remedy they might be using. As Dr Gerald Neuberg, associate clinical professor of medicine and director of the intensive care unit at New York Presbyterian Hospital's Allen Pavilion and a member of the advisory board for Quackwatch, points out:

> Alternative practitioners often make passionate claims that their patients feel better during treatment, and they probably do feel better, since the placebo effect is potent medicine. We all could build pretty successful practices by dispensing little else. But since controlled clinical trials generally have not been performed, the problem is how to distinguish the psychological or placebo benefits of the treatment from the actual intrinsic effects of the specific treatment.

One reason for the aforementioned lack of scientific research in CAM is that large, carefully controlled medical studies, are costly, and the pharmaceutical companies who develop and sell drugs, and who largely determine the direction and destiny of modern medicine, are utterly unmotivated to fund studies within the field of CAM. This is because the potential financial rewards that would be yielded from their investment would tend to be considerably less than those which result from the funding of treatments within the field of conventional medicine.

Because of the lack of solid scientific research in this area, readers are strongly advised always to consult their medical doctor before attempting to use any alternative, or CAM therapies.

Even if a doctor can't recommend a specific practitioner, he or she may be able to alert you to the possible risks and benefits before you try a treatment. It's especially important to involve your doctor if you are pregnant, have medical problems or take prescription medicine. And never stop or change your conventional treatment — such as the dose of your prescription medications — without talking to your doctor first.

Finally, be sure to keep your GP updated regarding any diets you adopt, and inform them if you are taking any vitamins, minerals or herbal supplements; since sometimes, these can interact dangerously with certain medications.

This book covers seven 'cutting-edge' therapies which are so unusual that many readers may find them unbelievable, but all of them are genuine, and each of them has attracted a modest, yet significant, number of followers. Pending the completion of clinically controlled trials it is very likely that some of the therapies in this book will have an extremely beneficial and revolutionary impact on mainstream medicine.

Chapter One: *Professor Nutt & Psychedelic Therapy*, is still undergoing scientifically controlled trials worldwide, and is yielding results which strongly suggest that certain psychedelics, used in a controlled, safe environment, could eventually be employed within the field of Psychiatry as an incredibly fast and effective treatment for depression, PTSD, addiction to alcohol and drugs, and also, as a highly effective psychotherapy for the terminally ill.

Chapter Two: *Dr Berceli's Trauma Therapy* taps into our genetically encoded capacity for dealing with trauma via a process known as Neurogenic Tremoring. Though still not in widespread use, it has proved itself to be so effective in alleviating the symptoms of Post-Traumatic Stress Syndrome, that it is now being employed by the US Military for the treatment of veterans of the Iraq and Afghanistan wars. It is also currently being tested in the USA on paramedics, firemen and police, with promising results. Currently it is attracting increasing interest among psychologists and psychiatrists specializing in trauma treatments.

Chapter Three: *Canine Diagnostics* relates the fascinating work of the charity 'Medical Detection Dogs', who train canines to smell the presence of early-stage cancer in patients, long before it can be detected by normal methods of diagnosis. It also provides Alert Assistance Canines as carers who can sense impending attacks in diseases such as brittle type 1 Diabetes which strikes its victims without warning. Though not yet in mainstream use, eminent medical specialists are deeply interested in exploring the diagnostic potential of this promising area.

Chapter Four: *Epley Omniax Vertigo Therapy* is still an unavailable medical approach in most countries but offers an impressive example of cutting-edge technology which has proved itself to be extremely effective in the diagnosis and treatment of various types of benign vertigo. Consequently, it has attracted the attention of a growing number of respected Otologists and Audiologists who are using it worldwide in a small number of private medical centres.

Chapter Five: *Helminth Therapy* provides a wealth of anecdotal evidence supporting its efficacy, but needs more clinically controlled trials to prove beyond any doubt that this incredible 'biotherapy' can successfully treat a variety of autoimmune disorders, which have failed to respond to conventional medicine. The results of various studies already suggest that in the not-too-distant future, this medical approach will prove to be a highly effective treatment for relieving sufferers from the symptoms of various autoimmune diseases.

Chapter Six: *Cutting Edge Apitherapy* has its roots in some of mankind's earliest approaches to medicine. Apitherapy, or Bee Venom Therapy (BVT) as it sometimes called, was used to treat joint problems in ancient Egypt, Greece, and China, and its medical applications were acknowledged by Hippocrates, the Greek physician known as the "Father of Medicine. However more recently, it has attracted some mainstream scientific interest following the results of a recent study published in 2009 in The Journal of Clinical Investigation. This showed that synthetic nanoparticles can be used successfully to deliver synthesized Mellitin, (bee-venom), in order to eliminate established tumours and pre-cancerous lesions in mice. These nanoparticles known as "nanobees" could eventually replace conventional therapy for certain types of cancer because the treatment has considerably fewer serious side-effects than does chemotherapy.

Chapter Seven: Finally, I predict that *Beer Spa Therapy*, though seemingly superficial and decadent, might, if used in moderation, actually turn out to bequeath significant benefits as a stress-release treatment for Epicureans – for those who are turned off by, and thus unwilling to adopt, more disciplined, less pleasurable approaches to stress reduction offered by systems such as meditation, Yoga and conventional fitness training. It is steadily growing in popularity in Germany and the Czech Republic and there is also one treatment center in the USA which offers this original approach to peace of mind.

CHAPTER ONE

PROFESSOR NUTT & PSYCHEDELIC THERAPY

This chapter is packed with fascinating information about one of the most controversial areas of psychiatry – psychedelic therapy. Research within this field of medicine has recently been resumed, having been banned for nearly half a century, and results of completed studies on the effects of psychedelics on war veterans with intractable PTSD and on subjects with treatment-resistant depression have been very promising. Currently, controlled studies on the efficacy of psychedelic treatment for depression are taking place at Johns Hopkins University School of Medicine in the USA and at the Neuropsychopharmacology Unit in the Division of Brain Sciences, at Imperial College London. The results so far suggest that within a decade, psychedelics could become a legal pharmacological treatment for depression and PTSD. What really surprised/shocked me was to discover toward the end of the chapter a list of numerous extremely well-known scientists, psychiatrists, philosophers, computer experts and authors who have experimented with these substances!

Dr Joakim Litzberg M.D. (Sweden)

There may be conventional-minded readers seeing the title of this chapter who will already be thinking *"Yet another crazy alternative therapy hits the market!"* In fact however, although prescribing psychedelic substances has always been a guaranteed way for a psychiatrist to lose his research funding or even his job, now scientists are starting to embrace the possibility that these drugs, though currently illegal, may be the key to treating a range of intractable illnesses, from depression to post-traumatic stress disorder.

Of course, psychedelic therapy is still in the research stage of its development, but current results suggest that in the not too distant future it may well be approved in the UK by The Medicine and Healthcare Products Regulatory Agency (MHRA) and in the USA by the FDA, as a tool for use in clinical psychology and psychiatry.

Professor David Nutt, British psychiatrist and director of the Centre for Neuropsychopharmacology at Imperial College, is at the forefront of this recent renaissance of scientific research. He is investigating the potential of psychedelic drugs, such as LSD, psilocybin and MDMA, as a means of treating addiction, depression and various other psychological and psychiatric disorders.

In January 2009, he become a centre of controversy when he published an article in the Journal of Psychopharmacology comparing the risks of horse riding (in which he found 1 person in 350 can expect acute harm) with ecstasy (1 in 10,000). In his article, titled *"Equasy: An overlooked addiction with implications for the current debate on drug harms"*, he wrote that *"equasy"*, short for *"Equine Addiction Syndrome"*, had caused 10 deaths and more than 100 road traffic accidents a year and that through hunting, it also led to "gatherings of users that often are associated with these groups engaging in violent conduct."

As such, Nutt claimed that 'Equine Addiction' should perhaps be classified as a *"class A drug given it appears more harmful than ecstasy."* He added that, *"Making riding illegal would completely prevent all these harms and would be, in practice, very easy to do"* and further, that there were plenty of other *"risky activities such as base jumping, climbing, bungee jumping, hang-gliding, motorcycling"* which were worse than *"many illicit drugs"*. This raises the question, *"of why society tolerates – indeed encourages – certain forms of potentially harmful behaviour but not others, such as drug use."*

On the basis of these comments, campaigners called for him to resign, suggesting that he was on a *"personal crusade"* to decriminalise the drug. In October 2009, he was finally dismissed as chair of the Government's Advisory Council on the Misuse of Drugs (a body of scientists, doctors, police officers and other experts who advise the Home Office).This was the day after he published a pamphlet containing a lecture he had given four months earlier, to the Centre for Crime and Justice Studies at King's College London.

The pamphlet ranked psychoactive substances in terms of damage, and concluded alcohol and tobacco to be considerably more harmful than illegal drugs such as LSD, cannabis and ecstasy, which are currently class-A drugs in the UK.

The following year, in November 2010, The Medical Journal Lancet - one of the world's oldest and most respected general medical journals - published their findings on drug risks. They concluded, as Nutt had, that overall, alcohol was the most harmful drug, with an overall harm score of 72, with heroin (55) and crack cocaine (54) in second and third places. Psilocybin came last, with an overall harm score of 6, and LSD came 18th with a score of 7.

Professor Nutt sees a parallel between the suppression of scientific research into the effects of psychedelic drugs, and the censorship of Galileo in the 17th century by the Catholic Church.

For over a hundred years, the church, ruled by their antiquated beliefs, prohibited Galileo and others from teaching or defending heliocentrism - the scientific observation that the Earth and planets revolve around the Sun at the centre of the solar system. Similarly, scientists and doctors today, are banned from studying many hundreds of drugs because of outdated United Nations charters dating back to the 1960s and 1970s.

Even in the U.S. where a small number of states have made medicinal cannabis available, it still remains illegal to research this drug without a special license from the Drug Enforcement Agency, and this costs so much and takes so long to acquire, that hardly any American researchers have one.

And this excessive regulation, from a health viewpoint, contrasts sharply and illogically with government attitudes toward legal pharmaceuticals which have proven to be considerably more harmful: The September 2016 issue of *Scientific American* pointed out that prescription painkilling opioids - such as Percocet and Fentanyl, which were implicated in the death of the pop star Prince – are used by millions of Americans each year, and overdoses of these legal drugs killed more than 165,000 Americans between 1999 and 2014, with the health and social costs of abusing such drugs totalling around $55 billion annually.

In contrast to this, between 1999 and 2010, in states which permitted the medical use of marijuana, there were 25% fewer opioid-related deaths, as compared with states where marijuana remained illegal. Moreover, the June issue of *Journal of Pain*, reports a survey which found that patients with chronic pain who began using medical marijuana, reduced their intake of opioid painkillers by half, and another study reported in the February 2016 issue of *Clinical Journal of Pain*, found that within seven months of taking medical cannabis, nearly half of opioid users entirely eliminated their intake of prescription opioids.

And yet in spite of the fact that it does not cause death and has such significant therapeutic potential, marijuana continues to be widely illegal in the U.S. and in Europe, while the prescribing of extremely dangerous opioid drugs still has not been banned or severely restricted. This state of affairs is testimony to the power and influence of government and giant pharmaceutical companies, who do not want to give up the vast profits they are making from these dangerous prescription drugs. And this behaviour also sits in stark contrast to the extreme paranoid reaction toward drugs such as MDMA which at its highest level of use, prior to it being made illegal, caused hundred deaths per year in the USA, in comparison with an average of 10,000 deaths caused annually by the aforementioned legal painkillers. Facts such as this are a constant inspiration to Professor Nutt and other pioneers who are currently involved in the fight to establish a healthier more balanced perspective on this entire situation.

Undeterred by his government dismissal, Nutt continued to fight valiantly for what he believed in, and in 2012, Imperial College London were awarded £550,000 by the UK Medical Research Council (MRC) to set-up a three-year clinical trial, headed by Nutt and his associate Dr Robin Carhart-Harris, to research the antidepressant potential of psilocybin (the psychoactive ingredient of all species of 'magic mushrooms').

Thanks to this grant, Nutt became the first scientist in the world to use various modern imaging modalities such as magnetic resonance imaging (MRI) to look at what parts of the brain are affected by psychedelics. His first study looked at how psilocybin affected the brain and recently he pioneered scans on volunteers after they had ingested LSD.

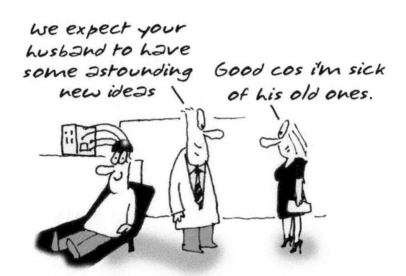

He and his team, which has also involved scientists from University of Bristol and Cardiff University, have since been funded by the Beckley Foundation, the Neuropsychoanalysis Foundation, The Multidisciplinary Association for Psychedelic Studies and the Heffter Research Institute.

In 2013 Professor Nutt was awarded the John Maddox Prize for Science, in recognition of the impact his thinking and actions have had globally in influencing evidence-based classification of drugs, and for his continued courage and commitment to rational debate, despite hostile opposition and public criticism.

Professor Colin Blakemore said:

The 2013 Prize recognises Professor Nutt's exceptional strength of character and his personal commitment to the open presentation of scientific evidence. In circumstances that would have humiliated and silenced most people...He took personal risk to his reputation in the name of sound science and in defending the right of researchers to present scientific opinion publicly...We need people like David Nutt to assert the independence of scientific advice and to inform the public when government policy departs from that advice.

The 60 volunteers in Nutts 2012 clinical study of psilocybin's effects on depression, had been classified as "treatment resistant" since they had previously failed to respond to two pharmaceutical treatments for depression, and his intention was to test 30 of these candidates with the drug and 30 with a placebo.

Nutt discovered that a single dose of psilocybin triggered a significant feeling of general wellbeing in his volunteer subjects that lasted several months. Professor Nutt's colleague, Carhart-Harris, believes that the psychedelic experience helps people by relaxing the grip of an overbearing ego and the rigid, habitual thinking it enforces. The sovereign ego can become a despot. This is perhaps most evident in depression, when the self turns on itself and uncontrollable introspection gradually shades out reality, a condition that Carhart-Harris calls *heavy self-consciousness.* This existential distress which increases even more, toward the end of life, is characterised by excessive self-reflection and an inability to escape the deepening grooves of negative thought. A single psychedelic experience — an intervention that Carhart-Harris calls *shaking the snow globe"* — can have the power to alter these patterns in a lasting way.

Psilocybin's antidepressant effects are therefore of exceptional importance, for as Dr Robin Carhart-Harris explains on his online website:

Depression is a serious global problem. It's the leading cause of disability worldwide, is linked to over half of all suicides, and affects some 350 million people...Around half of patients with depression do not respond to treatment with antidepressant medication and these medications, while effective in some patients, are associated with side-effects and need to be taken daily. Worse still, up to 20%

of people do not respond to any treatment at all and this leaves them isolated and with little hope…Our psilocybin research is focused on helping this group of 'treatment resistant' patients by offering an alternative option for their depression". Nutt claims: "This is potentially a revolution in the treatment of depression.

When Nutt infused psilocybin into the bloodstream of 30 volunteers who were laying inside magnetic resonance imaging (MRI) scanners, the changes in brain activity that were recorded, were exactly the opposite of what Nutt had predicted.

He had assumed that the 'mind-expanding' effects of these drugs were triggered by *increased* activity in the brain. In fact psilocybin functions by suppressing/reducing neuronal activity in parts of the brain that are known to constrain consciousness within the narrow boundaries of the normal waking state, by censoring and filtering out information in order to keep our experience of the world familiar and organized. Thus he concluded that it is the *deactivation* of these regions that enables the psychedelic experience.

- The following web address contains articles and videos relating the most recent work that has been carried out by Professor David Nutt and Dr Robin Carhart-Harris. http://psychedelic-science.org.uk/videos/

Fifty years earlier, in the 1960's, novelist and philosopher, Aldous Huxley, one of the western world's earliest and boldest 'psychonauts' (psychedelic explorer), had come to a similar realization after experimenting with mescaline.

He suggested what Nutt has now scientifically confirmed, that psychedelics temporarily suppress/inhibit activity in an area of the brain, whose normal function is to block from our conscious mind around 99.9% of the information that we are constantly picking up from our surroundings and the internal environment of our body, through cognitive processing, proprioception, and our five senses.

This part of the brain ensures that all this information is first fed directly to our unconscious mind. Here it is processed by a 'neurological editor' who instantaneously assesses and withholds from our conscious awareness, sensory and cognitive information that is not relevant for real-time decisions and other behaviour compatible with our current survival needs.

So although what we perceive of existence appears as if it is a 'live' feed from the sense organs, it is in fact a reconstructed, massively restricted, 'virtual' reality which our unconscious mind transmits to our conscious awareness a split second after it has 'edited out' data that it believes is either disadvantageous or unimportant for biological/psychological survival.

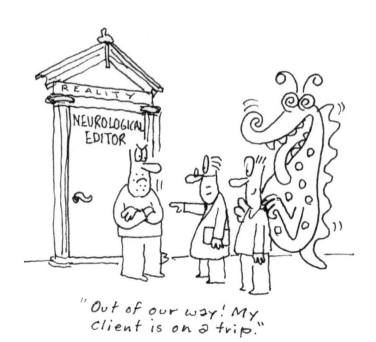

"Out of our way! My client is on a trip."

In 1965, Professor Dietrich Trincker, a German Physiologist from the University of Kiel explained this important fact in a summarization of decades of his work on the human brain:

> Of all the information that every second flows into our Brain, from our sensory organs, only a fraction arrives in our conscious: the ratio of the capacity of perception to the capacity of apparent perception is at best one million to one. This is to say that only one millionth of what our eyes see, our ears hear, and our other senses inform us about, appear in our conscious. It goes without saying that this newly verified fact has the greatest practical significance for all areas of human life.

For the sake of computer-proficient readers, we can look at this situation as a computer 'throughput' issue (the measure of how many units of information a system can process in a given amount of time).

Research conducted in 1962, ("Nachrichtenverarbeitung im Menschen") by Professor Karl Kupfmuller of the University of Darmstadt, claimed that between 10 million to 1000 million Bits per second of raw data is received by our sensory organs, and approximately 50% of this is retained in subliminal levels of memory, mostly sight data and sound data. He also demonstrated that only 40 bits per second of this information was made accessible to us - findings that were supported by investigations carried out by other researchers.

So it seems that in spite of the vast amount of data received through our senses by our unconscious mind, that the conscious mind does not receive, and cannot process more than the aforementioned 40 Bits per second of information. And we even edit out much of this information, because generally, we focus attention, only on that which is directly relevant to our survival, determined by our cultural conditioning, line of work, individual preferences, and various instincts such as the drive for sex and the innate genetic tendency instantly to notice dangers in the environment such as snakes.

It is clear, that there are obvious survival advantages to not having access to this vast amount of information stored in our subliminal mind, as can be seen in the case of rare individuals classed as 'savants'. One example is Daniel Tamett, who struggles to handle the simple needs of daily survival because he is constantly subjected to a massive onslaught of information.

Unlike Laurence Kim Peek, the incredible 'savant' who inspired the film *Rain Man*, Daniel Tamett does not suffer from congenital brain damage, he is mentally fairly normal, and his communication skills are adequate. He first became famous in 2014, on International Pi Day, when he recited from memory Pi to 22,514 decimal places in order to raise funds for the National Society for Epilepsy.

Daniel can calculate cube roots quicker than a calculator and has a rare form of synaesthesia which causes him to see integers (whole numbers) up to 10,000 as each having their own unique shapes, colour, texture and feel. This enables him to "see" the result of a math calculation, and he can "sense" whether a number is prime. For instance, Daniel has since drawn what pi looks like to him: a rolling landscape full of different shapes and colours.

In addition to all this, he speaks 11 languages, one of which is Icelandic, which Channel Five documentary challenged him to learn in a week, and exactly seven days later, Daniel was speaking the language reasonably fluently when interviewed on Icelandic television.

Most important of all, unlike all the other prodigious savants in the world, Daniel can actually explain to others how he achieves his amazing feats. This, according to Professor Allan Snyder, from the

Centre for the Mind at the Australian National University in Canberra, makes him a human 'Rosetta Stone', invaluable internationally to scientists exploring the potential of the human brain, by looking at the 'savant syndrome'.

However, because the 'subliminal editor' in Daniel's brain is allowing such a vast amount of data to reach his conscious mind, (thereby contributing to his amazing abilities), he is simultaneously so overwhelmed by this immense increase of accessible information, that he can't do simple things such as drive a car, wire a plug, or tell right from left. Even trips to the supermarket become a challenge: *"There's too much mental stimulus. I have to look at every shape and texture, every price and every arrangement of fruit and vegetables. So instead of thinking, 'What cheese do I want this week?' I'm just really uncomfortable."* And he never goes to stony beaches because *"there are too many pebbles to count".*

Aldous Huxley had experienced this same phenomenon when experimenting with psychedelics; he wrote that the mind is a *"reducing valve, eliminating far more reality than it admits to our conscious awareness, lest we be overwhelmed".* He concluded that in the normal human brain, the conscious mind is less a window on reality than a *"furious editor of it".* However Huxley also admonishes that the price we pay for our 'normal way of being' is that *"What comes out at the other end is a measly trickle of the kind of consciousness which will help us to stay alive..."* And when asked during an interview by *The Paris Review* (1960) to describe the experience of psychedelics, Huxley replied:

> It does help you to look at the world in a new way. And you come to understand very clearly the way that certain specially gifted people have seen the world. You are actually introduced into the kind of world that Van Gogh lived in, or the kind of world that

Blake lived in. You begin to have a direct experience of this kind of world while you're under the drug, and afterwards you can remember and to some slight extent recapture this kind of world, which certain privileged people have moved in and out of, as Blake obviously did all the time.

While one is under the drug one has penetrating insights into the people around one, and also into one's own life. Many people get tremendous recalls of buried material. A process which may take six years of psychoanalysis happens in an hour -- and considerably cheaper! And the experience can be very liberating and widening in other ways. It shows that the world one habitually lives in is merely a creation of this conventional, closely conditioned being which one is, and that there are quite other kinds of worlds outside. It's a very salutary thing to realize that the rather dull universe in which most of us spend most of our time is not the only universe there is. I think it's healthy that people should have this experience.

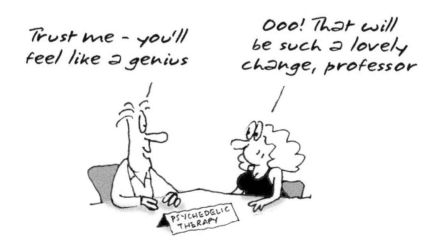

Huxley's final and possibly most important work *Island (1962)* - philosophically a blend of Mahayana Buddhism and Vedantic Hinduism - was the synthesis of decades of his intellectual and experiential research into spiritual mysticism and psychedelics which he saw as offering a powerful shortcut to liberation from the ego and freedom from the fear of death, but he also warns that the psychedelic experience is to be used only *"as an occasional treat"* as it is like banquets – *"they're too rich"* and require caterers. *"And that's precisely why there has to be meditation"* because *"For your everyday diet you have to do your own cooking."*

When Huxley was dying, his final words were: *"LSD, 100 micrograms I.M."* Huxley's wife Laura complied with his wishes, and the celebrated author of Brave New World crossed over into the White Light with Albert Hofmann's magic psychedelic saturating the synapses of his brain. In an extract from a letter to close friends, Laura describes the final moments prior to his death on November 22, 1963, which was assisted by intravenously injected LSD. The description begins at 9 a.m. when he entered a state of extreme agitation and restlessness that continued until he received LSD:

> …Aldous began to be so agitated, so uncomfortable, so desperate really…He wanted to be moved all the time… when I gave him the shot…a great relief came to us both… Now, the expression of his face was beginning to look as it did every time that he had the moksha medicine, when this immense expression of complete bliss and love would come over him…the ceasing of the breathing was not a drama at all, because it was done so slowly, so gently, like a piece of music just finishing in a *sempre piu* piano *dolcement*…all said that this was the most serene, the most beautiful death. Both doctors and nurse said they had never seen a person in similar physical condition going off so completely without pain and without struggle….

Faith in the therapeutic effects of psychedelics was already very evident in the 1950s through to the mid-1960s, when LSD was legal. Universities and hospitals, students and volunteers were paid for their willingness to test LSD, and hundreds of clinical trials of psychedelic drugs were carried out, with more than 1,000 scientific publications chronicling the ways that LSD could be used as an aid to make psychotherapy more effective. Psychiatrists were thrilled to have access to a drug that seemed to let the unconscious burst to the forefront, instantaneously dissolving the ego instead of slowly peeling it away layer by layer. Within the profession, word spread that LSD held the potential to cure alcoholism, schizophrenia, shell shock (now known as post-traumatic stress disorder), and a wide range of other problems. Between 1950 and 1965, a reported 40,000 people worldwide were tested or "treated" with LSD.

In the February 2015 issue of *The New Yorker* Magazine, Michael Pollan interviewed Stephen Ross, an associate professor of psychiatry at N.Y.U.'s medical school, who directs ongoing psilocybin trials, (he is also the director of the substance-abuse division at Bellevue). Ross explained that some of the best minds in psychiatry had received government funding to study the therapeutic potential of psychedelics. Between 1953 and 1973, the federal government spent $4million USD to fund 116 studies of LSD, involving more than 1700 subjects. (These figures don't include classified research.) And in the 1960's, LSD had been used successfully to treat alcoholics.

Similarly, in the 1970s, MDMA began to be used as a complement to talk therapy, and psychedelics in general, showed promise as a treatment for obsessive-compulsive disorder, addiction to alcohol and tobacco, depression and post-traumatic stress disorder (PTSD). But some of the most valuable and promising research that's been conducted with psychedelics has been in the area of treating the terminally ill.

Stephen Ross, related what for him was a landmark article in the field of psychedelic research. In July 2006, the *Journal of Psychopharmacology* published the results of a clinical trial carried out by Roland Griffiths at the Johns Hopkins University School of Medicine, which is regarded as the premier medical center in the USA. The article was titled *Psilocybin Can Occasion Mystical-Type Experiences Having Substantial and Sustained Personal Meaning and Spiritual Significance*. It concluded from the results that:

> When administered under supportive conditions, psilocybin occasioned experiences similar to spontaneously occurring mystical experiences that, over a year later, were considered by volunteers to be among the most personally meaningful and spiritually significant experiences of their lives and to have produced positive changes in attitudes, mood, altruism, behaviour and life satisfaction. In addition to possible therapeutic applications, the ability to prospectively produce mystical-type experiences should permit rigorous scientific investigations about their causes and consequences, and may provide novel information about the biological bases of moral and religious behaviour.

This study opened a gateway to a path in scientific research, that had been securely locked for more than three decades. Charles Grob at U.C.L.A., was the first to tread the path when he subsequently gained F.D.A. approval for a Phase I pilot study to assess the safety, dosing, and efficacy of psilocybin in the treatment of anxiety in cancer patients. Next came the Phase II trials, recently concluded in 2015 at both Hopkins and N.Y.U., involving higher doses and larger groups (29 at N.Y.U.; 56 at Hopkins). Thanks to this study Ross gained permission from NYU hospital in 2006 to test the psychedelic by guiding cancer patients through the experience. After receiving just a single dose of psilocybin, immediate and dramatic reductions in anxiety and depression were noted. People who had been palpably scared of death lost their fear and these improvements were sustained for at least six months. Ross asserted that, *"The fact that a drug given once can have such an effect for so long is an unprecedented finding. We have never had anything like it in the psychiatric field."*

Essential for ensuring a safe trip are three fundamentally important points:

- Set: the mental attitude of a would-be psychedelic voyager

- Setting: the surroundings in which a psychedelic substance is ingested

- Guides: *Two* guides who are experienced with non-ordinary states of consciousness who can help to mitigate challenges and channel insights

The following describes a typical guided psychedelic experience:

After the drug has been administered, subjects first report feeling significant fear and anxiety which subsides when they follow the advice of their 'guides', and surrender to the experience. Guides often choose to follow a set of instructions in a document created by Bill Richards, a Baltimore psychologist who, nearly fifty years ago, worked with the 'father' of psychedelic research, the eminent psychiatrist Stanislav Grof. Nowadays Bill Richards is deeply involved in training a new generation of psychedelic therapists. The instructions he compiled, are the fruit of experiences he accumulated from managing thousands of psychedelic sessions—and countless bad trips—during the nineteen-sixties and seventies.

The *"same force that takes you deep within will, of its own impetus, return you safely to the everyday world,"* his manual explains. Guides are instructed to reassure subjects that they'll never be left alone and that they should not worry about their bodies while journeying, since the guides will keep an eye on them. If you feel like you're *"dying, melting, dissolving, exploding, going crazy etc.—go ahead,"* embrace it: *"Climb staircases, open doors, explore paths, fly over landscapes."* And if you confront anything frightening, *"look the monster in the eye and move towards it. . . . Dig in your heels; ask, 'What are you doing in my mind?' Or, 'What can I learn from you?' Look for the darkest corner in the basement, and shine your light there."* Afterwards, the voyager is welcomed back and assisted with integrating into their life-situation any learning, insights, and mystical flashes that may have occurred.

The importance of well-trained guides cannot be overestimated, which is why since 2008, N.Y.U. has had a training program for guides directed by Jeffrey Guss, a co-principal investigator for the psilocybin trials.

Thanks to this type of stringent 'medical' training of guides, 'bad trips' that sometimes accompany the recreational use of psychedelics have not occurred during hundreds of sessions conducted over the past decade at places such as Imperial College London, N.Y.U. and Hopkins Medical center. It should be noted that the facilitators of psychedelic experiences carefully screen applicants to ensure that they are of a sufficiently sound mind for the treatment, and candidates are clearly informed of what the session can offer. This procedure helps to focus intentions, establish positive expectations, and dramatically increases the odds of a favourable outcome.

Volunteers in such trials often report that it is as though they are seeing their life situation from a distance, like looking through the wrong end of a telescope, so that events that previously had seemed traumatic and intolerable– including matters such as illness and death - now seem perfectly acceptable and manageable. Their descriptions are reminiscent of the "overview effect" described by astronauts who have glimpsed the earth from a great distance, an experience that some of them say permanently altered their priorities.

Roland Griffiths likens the therapeutic experience of psilocybin to a kind of *"inverse P.T.S.D."*—*"a discrete event that produces persisting positive changes in attitudes, moods, and behaviour, and presumably in the brain."* This likely explains the great success rate in removing or relieving the fear of death in terminal patients. Indeed, *"A high-dose psychedelic experience is death practice,"* according to Katherine MacLean, a former Hopkins psychologist. *"You're losing everything you know to be real, letting go of your ego and your body, and that process can feel like dying."* And yet you don't die.

Katherine MacLean hopes someday to establish a "psychedelic hospice," where the dying and their loved ones can use psychedelics to help them 'let go' and accept their life situation. *"If we limit psychedelics just to the patient, we're sticking with the old medical model,"* she said. *"But psychedelics are so much more radical than that. We are all terminal,"* Griffiths said. *"We're all dealing with death. This will be far too valuable to limit to sick people".*

- In the following video, Eddie Marritz, a cancer sufferer, relates his experience with Psilocybin at NYU:
  http://www.newyorker.com/tech/elements/
  video-magic-mushrooms-healing-trip?intcid=mod-latest

Stanislav Grof saw the immense value of psychedelics as a therapy for the dying, when he and colleagues at Spring Grove State Hospital in Baltimore carried out clinically controlled trials on terminally ill patients from 1967 - 1972, using LSD combined with psychotherapy. The results showed that this treatment could alleviate, in therapy-resistant terminally ill patients, symptoms of depression, tension, anxiety, sleep disturbances, psychological withdrawal, and even severe physical pain that was resistant to opiates. It also improved communication between the patients and their loved ones. *"Psychedelics could be for psychiatry what the microscope is for biology or the telescope for astronomy."* (Stanislav Grof, 1975).

Psychiatric researcher Rick Strassman's human trials with the synthetic psychedelic DMT (also found naturally in the brain) may indicate - by mimicking some important aspects of the near-death experience - the type of biochemical/psychological changes that occur in the brain when we're dying. Strassman hypothesizes that, *"DMT levels rise with the stress associated with near-death experiences, and mediate some of the more "psychedelic features of this state."*

The 'psychonaut' Timothy Leary must have been very aware of the close affinity between 'tripping' and dying, since the book he wrote as a guide for people having a psychedelic experience, was based upon the Tibetan Buddhist text, *Tibetan Book of the Dead*. In other words, it appears that the chemicals in certain psychedelics may be closely related to neurotransmitters naturally produced when we are close to death, whose effects are remarkably similar to those described during a psychedelic trip.

This suggests that in the case of terminally ill patients, including those who are right on the verge of death, the use of psychedelics may well be perfectly compatible with their needs both from a psychotherapeutic point of view as well as at deep physiological levels.

Unfortunately however, in spite of the extremely promising results arising from Stanislav Grof's investigation of the therapeutic potential of LSD so many years ago; the entire area of psychedelic research was subsequently abandoned and only recently recommenced. This was due to the widespread use and abuse of psychedelics as recreational drugs by the 'flower power' culture, which resulted in LSD being regulated almost out of existence in the US in 1970 and by the UN in 1971. According to Professor Nutt, scientists are only just catching up with *"50 years of censorship"*.

But psychedelic researchers are now becoming increasingly optimistic regarding the future of psychedelic therapy, in the light of increasing numbers of promising studies.

Importantly, an article in the March 2015 issue of *Scientific American* suggests the possibility that psychedelics may soon be exonerated from their bad reputation, something which has been prevalent for so many years. Two recent studies mentioned in the article, clearly suggest that widespread reports in mainstream news of *"acid casualties"*, from the 1960's to present times, have been massively exaggerated and have contributed to long-held fears in our culture that psychedelics frequently lead to psychosis and suicide.

The first of these studies was conducted by clinical psychologists Pål-Ørjan Johansen and Teri Suzanne Krebs, at the Norwegian University of Science and Technology in Trondheim. Their conclusions were the result of data analysed from a random sample of more than 135,000 of the general population, whom had taken part in surveys from 2008 to 2011, conducted by the US National Survey on Drug Use and Health (NSDUH).

They noted that 14% of the participants in the survey described themselves as having used at some point in their lives one or more of the three 'classic' psychedelics: LSD, psilocybin (the active ingredient in so-called magic mushrooms) and mescaline (found in the peyote and San Pedro cacti). In spite of this, the prevalence of 11 indicators of mental-health problems such as schizophrenia, psychosis, depression, anxiety disorders and suicide attempts was not, statistically speaking, significantly higher in this section than among the group of non-users in the survey.

Krebs explains the fundamental cause for the irrational paranoia in society toward psychedelics: *"since psychotic disorders are relatively prevalent in our society, affecting about one in 50 people, correlations have often been mistaken for causations"*. Their paper appeared in the March 2015 issue of the *Journal of Psychopharmacology*.

The second of these two recent studies, published in the same Journal, analysed the responses of 190,000 NSDUH respondents from 2008 to 2012. It also found that the classic psychedelics were not associated with adverse mental-health outcomes, but most importantly, it further discovered that people who had used LSD and psilocybin had *lower* lifetime rates of suicidal thoughts and suicidal attempts. *"We are not claiming that no individuals have ever been harmed by psychedelics,"* says author Matthew Johnson, an associate professor in the Behavioural Pharmacology Research Unit at Johns Hopkins University in Baltimore, Maryland. *"Anecdotes about acid casualties can be very powerful—but these instances are rare,"* he says (and thus not considered "statistically significant").

These landmark observations challenge public fears that the ingestion of psychedelic drugs, such as LSD, strongly predisposes users to various mental-health conditions including psychosis and suicidal thoughts.

Indeed, Professor Nutt thinks that the government should have a far more lenient attitude towards drugs in general. Although he acknowledges the necessity of criminalizing extremely harmful drugs like heroin and crack, he asserts that placing softer drugs such as cannabis in the same category as these, has allowed dealers to monopolize and saturate the market with super-strong varieties of the drug. One example being 'skunk', which has been shown by a King's College London investigation to cause 25% of new cases of psychosis.

The banning of such drugs also contributes to the widespread, steadily increasing alcohol abuse in society:

> "We need to accept the fact that most people like to change the way they feel," Professor Nutt said. "Most people use alcohol. My view is that any drug that is less harmful than alcohol should be made available in some kind of regulated fashion because that will reduce the harms of alcohol."

Queen Victoria's physician understood the value of tincture of cannabis, which the monarch apparently used to reduce the pain of menstrual periods and childbirth. Yet now it is denied to patients in the UK suffering from neurological disorders and cancer. Why?

According to Professor Nutt, when alcohol prohibition was repealed, in order to maintain his celebrity status and powerful position, Harry Anslinger, who had headed the prohibition enforcement team, enlisted the support of newspaper magnate, William Randolph Hearst, to create a web of lies. This included the *"invasion of marijuana-smoking Mexican men assaulting white women"* that inflamed public hysteria toward the use of marijuana, causing it to be banned in the US and subsequently the rest of the world via the first UN convention on narcotic drugs in 1961.

This same theme of arousing a paranoia of drugs by inciting a fear of the "other people" who use them continued with the stigmatisation of black Americans in the 1950's who were accused of heroin use. Then, in the 1960s, psychedelics and hippies became the target because they opposed the Vietnam War.

> Psychedelics are illegal because they dissolve opinion structures and culturally laid down models of behaviour and information processing. They open you up to the possibility that everything you know is wrong. (Terence McKenna)

A more recent example of this trend can be seen in the UK, where the right wing press incited a hate campaign fuelled by prejudice, and camouflaged by a smokescreen of fabricated health concerns, against peace-loving young people, which resulted in MDMA and raves being banned, in spite of the fact that most police felt completely unthreatened by MDMA users, who were generally very friendly, unlike those attending alcohol-fuelled events.

Nutt says that this ban on MDMA has resulted in considerably *more dangerous* and completely *untested* legal highs coming on to the market, that have been responsible for a considerably *greater* number deaths. Writing for The Guardian, he asserted:

> The emergence of the more toxic PMA following the so-called 'success' in reducing MDMA production is just one of many examples of how prohibition of one drug leads to greater harm from an alternative that is developed to overcome the block.

PMA is similar to MDMA (the chemical in ecstasy) but is *far* more poisonous, and because the effects take longer to be felt, users are more likely to overdose because they think they have not taken a sufficient amount.

Similarly, statistics show that deaths from cocaine and amphetamine *decreased* by up to 40% because many switched over to the legal high 'mephedrone'. However it was subsequently banned in 2010, in spite of extremely low death statistics in comparison with most other drugs, and cocaine deaths rose again to their pre-mephedrone levels.

This prohibition of mephedrone was due to yet another relentless campaign by politicians siding with certain youth-hating newspapers. This created a situation that Professor Nutt compared to the rise in demand for more poisonous hooch after alcohol was prohibited in the US during the 1920s, and to the rise in production and injecting of heroin after smoking opium was banned.

So each time the younger generation discovers a thoroughly tested legal high, such as MDMA, which allows them to enjoy altered states of consciousness without risking a criminal record, the newspapers fight to get it banned. And in the case of MDMA, this is in spite of evidence that it dramatically reduces alcohol abuse among users, and though dangerous with prolonged use, and lethal when overdosed, statistically speaking, is considerably less dangerous than drugs such as alcohol, heroin and crack cocaine, not to mention the numerous, far more dangerous legal highs that former MDMA users take in its place. It is interesting to note that this illogical, ineffective tactic is covertly supported by the alcohol industry who oppose any substance that could reduce alcohol consumption or challenge its monopoly of recreational drugs. And yet, alcohol ranks among the top five causes of death in EU nations, with the Government classifying it as the leading cause of premature death in the UK among men aged 16 to 54. It shortens our lives in many ways: liver disease, a dozen forms of cancer, elevated blood pressure, strokes, heart attacks, increased risk of dementia, car crashes, domestic abuse and crime; and as Nutt points out, "The health costs amount to £3billion a year."

In stark contrast to the damaging effects of alcohol, many are becoming increasingly hopeful and optimistic that psychedelics may become the 'saviour' of mankind. The late Robert Muller was Assistant Secretary General of the United Nations for 40 years and is regarded by many as "the philosopher of the United Nations". He was also the winner of numerous prestigious awards including: UNESCO Prize for Peace Education; Albert Schweitzer International Prize for the Humanities; Eleanor Roosevelt Man of Vision Award; and the Goi Peace Award 2003, and he authored numerous books, including *New Genesis: Shaping a Global Spirituality*. Muller was convinced that underlying conflicts between nations were invariably rooted in religious conflict and he believed that the mystical experience of unity could become the antidote to fundamentalism if genuine mystics from the different religions were to gather together to teach peace. After viewing evidence which demonstrated that psychedelics can help catalyse spiritual, mystical experiences with lasting beneficial effects, and in agreement with Einstein's viewpoint that *"A new type of thinking is essential if mankind is to survive,"* Muller helped Rick Doblin, Ph.D., founder and director of the Multidisciplinary Association for Psychedelic Studies (MAPS)) to gain permission from the government to resume psychedelic research.

And his help yielded results, which proved to be a real blessing for war veterans such as Tony Macie who, like tens of thousands of other veterans from the wars in Afghanistan and Iraq, came back from duty in 2007, diagnosed with post-traumatic stress disorder (PTSD).

Macie went to the Department of Veterans' Affairs (VA) *"on and off"* and tried the standard therapy, but says the care he received at the VA – anti-anxiety and anti-depressants combined with therapy, and painkillers for his back – only made him numb. He eventually became addicted to Oxycodone. *"You're not dead, you're not alive,"* he said.

In 2011 Macie volunteered to take part in a trial, organized by the Multidisciplinary Association for Psychedelic Studies (MAPS). Founded by Rick Doblin, Ph.D., it was in the second phase of clinical trials, using psychotherapy in conjunction with pure MDMA. This was the key ingredient in the illegal drug ecstasy, which in laboratory studies, has been proven sufficiently safe for human consumption when taken a limited number of times in moderate doses.

- This study, as well as all previous and ongoing research studies, can be located at the MAPS website:http://www.maps.org/

The medical trial treated U.S. veterans, firefighters, and police officers with chronic, treatment-resistant PTSD. The results were remarkable: after treatment, 83 percent of the subjects no longer met the criteria for the diagnosis of PTSD, and a long-term follow-up of these volunteers revealed that overall benefits were maintained for an average of 3.8 years.

The results were published in the Journal of Psychopharmacology. *"As far as the percentage of people that have these really robust responses, I've never seen anything like it,"* said Dr. Michael Mithoefer, the study's principal investigator. *"It's the most promising drug I've come across as a psychiatrist."*

Mithoefer states that MDMA works by weakening the grip of traumatic memories.

People that are traumatized and then develop PTSD are trapped in a way where the past is always present…The MDMA reduces their fear of these memories. Suddenly, they can revisit the trauma without being overwhelmed but still with a clear memory.

MDMA allows patients to recall the painful past, while excising the visceral fight-or-flight reaction that normally accompanies traumatic memories. *"They reconsolidate, or restore the memory, in a different way that is not connected to the fear".*

Rick Doblin explains that unlike antidepressants, patients given psychedelic-assisted therapy don't need to be medicated for an extended period of time:

> It's not meant to be like a daily medication that changes people's biochemistry…People only get MDMA three times in our treatment process. People only get psilocybin or LSD a few times. The goal is to actually cure the problem unlike most medications for mental illnesses which are often taken daily for years, and sometimes forever.

Mithoefer was by Macie's side when he took his first dose of MDMA. He was given an eye mask and headphones to listen to music. He lay down and waited for the drug to take effect. Macie describes his experience:

> It was just like a paradigm shift. The medication kicked in and I went from feeling anxious to feeling nothing, just complete relaxation…I felt like I had an ache in my chest and it was just released. It was a wave of not pleasure – but relief – that I could let this memory go…I still remembered it, but was just moving on from it.

Macie says a single session of MDMA-assisted psychotherapy accomplished what four years of conventional therapy and medications at the VA could not:

> What it did was allow me to address things without judgment. I was able to think about the war. I was able to think about when I got back. It gave me a lot of closure. And it also gave me a lot of power to live my life and put me back in control.

It's been four years since the trial and Macie remains free from all medication. If all goes well, Rick Doblin predicts that MDMA will become a prescription medication in 2021. But Macie emphasizes that this waiting period is too long for the veterans currently suffering what he experienced, especially, he says, when an average of *"22 veterans are committing suicide every day"*.

Currently however there is one country in the world – Switzerland - where it *is* possible to receive medically supervised LSD and MDMA psychedelic therapy, or at least, a variation of it known as Psycholytic Therapy.

Psycholytic Therapy is the term used in reference to entheogen-enhanced psychoanalysis. Broadly speaking, the term entheogen is used to refer to psychoactive drugs that are used for the purpose of their religious, spiritual or psychological benefits rather than for recreational purposes. Psycholytic therapy is a term first used by Stanislav Grof in 1976 to describe his successful use of moderate doses of LSD to treat a wide range of neurotic and psychotic psychopathologies.

Psycholoytic therapy, as described by Stanislav Grof, differs from many other approaches to psychedelic therapy. It involves an extensive preparatory stage where the therapist administers "drug free" psychotherapy in order to establish boundaries, client orientation, and a healthy and trusting therapeutic relationship. This is followed by several sessions of moderate dose LSD therapy, starting with 100 micrograms and increasing until an "optimum dosage" is determined. According to Grof:

> Criterion for the optimum dose were an adequate depth of self-exploration, the overcoming of important psychological defenses, the emergence of sufficient amount of unconscious material, and, at the same time, the ability to maintain a good therapeutic content.

During the experience, as with other forms of psychedelic therapy, the therapist stays with the patient (the experiencer). In the case of the typical LSD experience, this can require a commitment of between twelve and sixteen hours. Following this, Grof advises patients not be left without supervision. In between sessions, drug free de-briefing and analysis sessions are provided and throughout the course of psycholytic therapy, detailed clinical records are kept.

In 1988, the Swiss Federal Office for Public Health granted Dr Peter Gasser and four other psychiatrists' permission to implement and research the use of LSD and MDMA in their private psychotherapeutic practice, despite the global ban. All five were members of the Swiss Medical Society for Psycholytic Therapy, a society founded in 1985 with the goal of training qualified therapists to use psycholytic psychotherapy as a psychotherapeutic method in their practice. Three of the initial five therapists, Dr. Marianne Bloch, Dr. Jurai Styk and Dr. Samuel Widmer, worked all five and a half years with drug-assisted therapy until 1993 when all psychedelic research was once again forbidden.

However, in 2007, Dr Gasser sponsored by MAPS, finally gained approval from the Swiss Ministry of Health to use LSD to treat patients with cancer or other life-threatening diseases who struggled with end-of-life anxiety. After seven years of research, the study was published in November 2014 under the name *"LSD-assisted psychotherapy for anxiety associated with a life-threatening disease: A qualitative study of acute and sustained subjective effects."* This was the first controlled trial of the drug in the 21st century.

Following this successful study, Gasser successfully applied to the Swiss government for "compassionate use" authorization to include LSD in his therapy practice.

> The good thing with the compassionate use is I am not restricted to cancer patients; I can apply to treat patients with any kind of problems if I have a good theory about what LSD would help with and why exactly LSD would work. If the Swiss government agrees, I'm granted permission to use it.

Gasser continues to administer the drug to patients today, in both individual and group settings. Gasser's therapy room is lined with comfortable couches and floor cushions, a statue of Buddha and a nice stereo system that no doubt is integrated into his guided trips. He is the only person in the world with this permission to administer LSD as a treatment in private therapeutic practice, though a colleague and friend of his, Dr. Peter Oehen has also been granted permission for the "compassionate use" of MDMA.

The treatments take place in a meditative setting with candles, flowers and blinds to dim the daylight, and there is just the patient and two therapists: Gasser and a female colleague. There are no eyeshades or headphones, though music guides the experience together with intermittent periods of silence of equal length, which allows the process to develop and deepen. During the session, clients according to their individual preference, keep their eyes open or closed, though most alternate between the two. They speak whenever inclined, though they are encouraged to postpone any desire for lengthy discussion until the following day which allows for a more profound experience.

LSD has also proven to be dramatically effective in boosting creativity. The most extensive and respected scientific study on its effects in this area was completed in 1966. It was headed by Dr James Fadiman, who had for several years been exploring how psychedelics in general—and LSD in particular—could safely augment psychotherapy, addiction treatment, creative endeavours, and spiritual growth. His interest in this field of research had been inspired in 1961 following a personal psilocybin experience provided by his friend, Harvard professor Richard Alpert (Ram Dass). Since this time he had been convinced that humans would be able to live in far greater harmony if they could access the type of cosmic consciousness provided by such experiences, and he became deeply committed to achieving this objective.

Fadiman was a researcher at the International Foundation for Advanced Study (IFAS), a privately funded facility dedicated to psychedelic drug research in Menlo Park, California, which had legally dispensed LSD for the previous five years.

The organization had been founded in 1960 by Myron Stolaroff, a graduate of Electrical Engineering from Stanford University. He was also an eminent researcher and design engineer who had co-designed the Ampex Model 200A reel-to-reel tape recorder that revolutionized the radio and recording industries. However, after personally experiencing LSD Stolaroff devoted the rest of his life to researching the potential beneficial effects of LSD, mescaline, and other drugs, on psychotherapy and creativity. He claimed that:

> In one day I learned more about reality and who we are as human beings than I had ever imagined before. I considered it the most important discovery I would ever make and that there was nothing more important for me to do than to realize the entire potential LSD offered.

The final day of Fadiman's research project investigating LSD's capacity to enhance creativity, is a highly memorable one, because at approximately 10 a.m., a courier delivered an express letter to the receptionist, who in turn quickly relayed it to Fadiman and the other researchers. They were to stop administering LSD, by order of the U.S. Food and Drug Administration. Effective immediately, dozens of other private and university-affiliated institutions had received similar letters that day. However, Fadiman's final four test subjects involved in the study had already been dosed at 9:30 am, prior to the arrival of the letter, so cooperation with the FDA edict was literally an impossibility. The results of this experiment were added later to those of the twenty two other men who had taken part in this same IFAS research project over the course of the preceding year.

Scientists from Stanford, Hewlett-Packard, a commercial artist, a furniture designer and an electronics engineer were among the volunteers. Each test subject brought three highly technical problems from their respective fields that they'd been unable to solve for several months. Donning earphones and eye masks, they settled down into comfy couches, waiting for their government-approved dose of LSD to kick in, while Dr. James Fadiman simultaneously commenced a recording of Beethoven's "Symphony No. 6 in F Major, Op. 68."

They had each taken a relatively low dose of acid, 100 micrograms, and the intention was that when the effects of the LSD would be fully active they would remove the earphones and eye masks and attempt to find solutions to their hitherto insoluble problems, thereby ascertaining the effects of LSD on creative and analytical thinking. Any creative output derived while under the influence of the substance, would be scrutinized by departmental chairs, zoning boards, review panels, corporate clients, and the like, thus providing a real-world, unbiased yardstick for their results.

After the LSD-enhanced problem-solving sessions, the volunteers, some of the best and brightest minds in their fields, were all in agreement that LSD had been absolutely invaluable in helping them to find solutions to their seemingly intractable problems. And the aforementioned establishment assessing them, agreed with their conclusions.

Douglas Engelbart, who invented the computer mouse, along with his creation of the "copy and paste" technique, was one of many engineers who participated in this IFAS study on the connection between LSD and enhanced creativity. Of the remaining 25 men who participated, a number of them embraced innovations that surfaced in the months following their LSD experiences. This included a mathematical theorem for NOR gate circuits, a conceptual model of a photon, a technical improvement of the magnetic tape recorder, a space probe experiment designed to measure solar properties, and a linear electron accelerator beam-steering device.

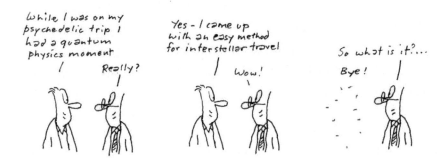

Yet, in spite of the amazing results published by Fadiman, he and his colleagues were forced to close all further research studies into the effects of LSD, as it was subsequently banned by the FDA.

At a congressional subcommittee later in the same year, Sen. Robert F. Kennedy grilled FDA regulators about this ban on LSD research: *"Why, if they were worthwhile six months ago, why aren't they worthwhile now?"* For him, the ban was personal too: His wife, Ethel, had received LSD-augmented therapy in Vancouver. *"Perhaps to some extent we have lost sight of the fact that it"*—Sen. Kennedy was referring specifically to LSD here—*"can be very, very helpful in our society if used properly."*

When Carhart-Harris was asked his opinion as to why LSD was prohibited, in spite of its proven beneficial effects, he had a surprising answer: *"the Vietnam war"*. He explains:

> Young Americans realised they didn't want to fight any more. That brought a huge tension into society. So they had to create reasons for banning the drug. Everyone knew the arguments were totally specious. But no one stood up.

Carhart-Harris has a further explanation:

> Psychedelics are scary because they reveal the mind, and people are scared of their own minds. They're scared of the human condition, really.

In Johns Hopkins' ongoing program of psilocybin research, scientists have treated over 150 volunteers in 350 drug-trial sessions. Although many participants experienced some type of anxiety reaction while on the drug, none of them reported lasting harm, and 70% rated the experience as one of the top five most meaningful events of their lives.

The popular belief that LSD is extremely dangerous and causes damage to the brain, resulting in severe psychological disorders, and that its addictive properties are not far behind those of heroin, is clearly highly suspect, especially in light of the aforementioned results of the study conducted by Johansen and Krebs which analysed data from the US National Survey on Drug Use and Health involving 135,000 and then 190,000 respondents; and especially when one considers the fact that some of the greatest writers, artists, scientists, mathematicians and inventors in history, credit LSD for enhancing their creative or scientific realizations.

Indeed, when LSD became popular in the 1960s, its influence on creative expression was indisputable, as new inventions and expressions of creativity dramatically increased in fields such as architecture, technology, music, painting and fashion.

The following portfolio of influential scientists, inventors and artists who were inspired by LSD, suggests that the substance allows us to forge deeper relationships with the natural world and that it can inspire us to explore and expand the limits of our imagination, resulting in creative expression in a multitude of different areas of life. More importantly, LSD and other psychedelics can awaken our spiritual heart, opening portals to a profound sense of connection with all living beings on earth, and in the universe as whole.

PLEASE NOTE: If the information I have provided on psychedelics has inspired you, the reader, to consider experimenting with these substances, then you are strongly urged *not* to do so, unless the experience is recommended, and fully supervised, by a qualified clinical psychologist or psychiatrist who has been formally trained and legally licensed to engage in the therapeutic application of psychedelics.

The psychedelic experience is extremely inappropriate for certain individuals and this is why it is crucial to be assessed by a psychiatrist or clinical psychologist trained in their use, prior to trying out this approach to therapy. In addition, if psychedelics are taken in the wrong setting, or in the wrong state of mind, or if they are used in in the absence of appropriate supervision, they can potentially be extremely harmful or dangerous, even if you happen to be an appropriate candidate for this type of treatment.

Finally, I would also like to make my position clear to the reader, with regard to the recreational use of other illegal substances:

Drugs of any sort should *only* ever be taken, if they are recommended and strictly supervised by a psychiatrist, doctor or clinical psychologist who can determine whether or not there is a genuine medical need for a particular substance.

For instance, in the USA, in more than 25 states, marijuana can be appropriately, and legally prescribed by doctors to relieve the symptoms of various illnesses including: Multiple Sclerosis, Muscular Dystrophy, Glaucoma, Nausea (e.g. from side-effects of chemotherapy) rheumatoid arthritis, epileptic seizures, Muscle Spasms, Tourette Syndrome, Brain and Spinal Cord injury, and Lupus.

However, there are numerous reasons for *not* using marijuana if one has no valid medical justification:

Marijuana contains nearly 50% more of the cancer-irritant benzopyrene than does tobacco, and it deposits in the lungs four times as much cancer-causing tar. It saps energy, producing feelings of deep fatigue, and damages physical coordination and reaction time thereby diminishing driving and other psychomotor skills. Marijuana seriously impairs cognitive performance since it damages memory and concentration, temporarily producing symptoms that are reminiscent of advanced dementia - 60% of student marijuana users report that they often forget what a conversation is about before it has ended. There is no doubt that in many people, this drug also dramatically reduces motivation and ambition, because it numbs the emotions, causing users to avoid dealing with problems since they become indifferent to their life circumstances and also lack the energy and desire needed to make positive changes.

Some Famous Scientists, Inventors and Important pioneers who used LSD:

It seems appropriate to preface this section of the chapter with the following observations by Albert Einstein and by Albert Hoffman, the discoverer of LSD:

Einstein argued that *"Man"* suffers from an *"optical delusion of consciousness"* because:

> He experiences himself, his thoughts and feelings as something separated from the rest…The most beautiful thing we can experience is the mysterious…It is the source of all true art and science. He to whom this emotion is a stranger, who can no longer pause to wonder and stand rapt in awe, is as good as dead: His eyes are closed.

Albert Hofmann discussing LSD for his 100th birthday speech:

In 1938, Hoffman, then a 32-year-old Swiss chemist, synthesized *Lysergic Acid Diethylamide-25*, popularly called LSD, while experimenting with fungus in search of a stimulant for the central nervous system. It wasn't until 1943 that he discovered its psychoactive properties by accident, when he unintentionally consumed some of his own compound, and then on many further occasions when he intentionally ingested it:

> Of greatest significance to me has been the insight that I attained as a fundamental understanding from all of my LSD experiments: what one commonly takes as 'the reality,' including the reality of one's own individual person, by no means signifies something fixed, but rather something that is ambiguous—that there is not

only one, but that there are many realities, each comprising also a different consciousness of the ego…I became aware of the wonder of creation, the magnificence of nature…It gave me an inner joy, an open mindedness, a gratefulness, open eyes and an internal sensitivity for the miracles of creation…I think that in human evolution it has never been as necessary to have this substance LSD. It is just a tool to turn us into what we are supposed to be.

Francis Crick (1916-2004)

The fact that psychedelics have changed the course of science and our understanding of existence is indisputable, and one of the best examples of this is seen in the case of the molecular biologist and physicist. Often referred to as the "father of modern genetics," Crick was a fan of Aldous Huxley's work *The Doors of Perception*, which narrated the authors experiments with psychedelics. Crick had told a Cambridge associate, Dick Kemp, that he had perceived the double-helix shape of DNA while on LSD. The event took place in 1953, when he apparently burst through the front door of his home in Cambridge while 'tripping', and excitedly described to his wife Odile, his vision of two spirals intertwining and twisting in opposite directions from one another. Odile, an artist, was inspired to draw what became the very first image of the double helix structure of DNA. Subsequently, in 1962, Crick and two associates were awarded the Nobel Prize for their landmark discoveries in this area.

Crick never made it a secret that he experimented with the drug, and admitted that prior to his discovery, he and various colleagues had been ingesting periodically small doses of the drug to boost creative thinking.

Kary Banks Mullis

Awarded the Nobel Prize for Chemistry in 1993, Mullis is credited with the invention of PCR (Polymerase Chain Reaction), although in fact, he did not *invent* it but improved it to the extent that it revolutionized the field of biomedical research.

PCR is a biochemical technology used to amplify a few copies of a piece of DNA and generate thousands of copies of a particular DNA sequence, a technique that helps in isolating, studying and testing the DNA in depth.

In a Q&A interview published in the September 1994, issue of California Monthly, Mullis said:

> Back in the 1960s and early '70s I took plenty of LSD. A lot of people were doing that in Berkeley back then. And I found it to be a mind-opening experience. It was certainly much more important than any courses I ever took.

During a symposium held for centenarian Albert Hofmann, Hofmann revealed that Kary Mullis confessed to him that LSD had helped him develop PCR. Some years later, in an interview for BBC's Psychedelic Science documentary, Mullis pondered:

> Would I have invented PCR if I hadn't taken LSD? I seriously doubt it. I could sit on a DNA molecule and watch the polymers go by. I learnt that partly on psychedelic drugs.

Steve Jobs

Not long after he passed away from pancreatic cancer, it soon became widely known that Steve Jobs, co-founder of Apple and arguably the most innovative pioneer in the personal computer revolution, had taken LSD around 15 times between 1972 and 1974. Jobs credits his outside-the-box perspective to LSD which bestowed on him an entirely different vision of existence that inspired a lot of Apple's product inventions and success:

> Throughout that period of time I used the LSD approximately ten to fifteen times…I would ingest the LSD on a sugar cube or in a hard form of gelatine. I would usually take the LSD when I was by myself. I have no words to explain the effect the LSD had on me, although, I can say it was a positive life-changing experience for me and I am glad I went through that experience…Taking LSD was a profound experience, one of the most important things in my life. LSD shows you that there's another side to the coin, and you can't remember it when it wears off, but you know it. It reinforced my sense of what was important—creating great things instead of making money, putting things back into the stream of history and of human consciousness as much as I could.

In his biography he stated that the people he knew and worked with, including his wife, were incapable of truly understanding certain aspects of who he was, because they had not taken psychedelics. It was known that during interviews, he would sometimes ask potential Apple employees if they had ever done LSD.

Mark Pesce

In 1993 Mark Pesce - inventor, writer, entrepreneur, educator and broadcaster - was hired by Steve Job's Computer Corporation Apple as a consulting engineer, to develop interfaces between Apple and IBM networking products. A year later in 1994, he co-invented VRML, a

3D interface to the World Wide Web. Pesce convinced the industry to accept the new protocol as a standard for desktop virtual reality.

When interviewed by researchers from MAPS, who asked Mark Pesce: How have psychedelics affected your creative process? He replied:

> I'm not sure that I'd be doing any of the work that I'm doing now. I don't know. I think I'd probably be some silly software engineer working in New England, unenlightened and bored with life, without psychedelics. I can almost guarantee that. My use of psychedelics and my intellectual career essentially began synonymously somewhere in the first or second year of college. And so there was an opening up that came from the psychedelic experience…it gave me a magnetic center -- that's what the Gurdjieffians would call it… And from that, what I had to do was just follow where that center would take me, and listen to it. And the times in my life when I've gotten fucked up are the times when I haven't done that. By the time I got a little bit older, I was into what Joseph Campbell would call "following your bliss." Well, my bliss was revealed through the psychedelic experience. It wasn't achieved through the psychedelic experience, but it was revealed through the psychedelic experience.

MAPS: Do you ever use psychedelics for problem-solving tasks? Where you have a specific question in mind, and then you take psychedelics in search of an answer?

> They've certainly been facilitators or catalysts for that. The most striking example is all the cyberspace protocols that came to me. I mean "wham," it came to me like that, and I just saw them. I got the big picture, but the big picture said, "Okay, well you know roughly how to make it work. Now you have to go in and do the detail, right?" I spent three years doing that detail work, and

out of that detail work came VMRL, and some stuff which you'll probably still see in a couple of years.

Ralph Abraham

Prominent mathematician, known for his lectures on "Chaos" theory, Ralph Abraham is Professor Emeritus of Mathematics at University of California. He is also a well-known author who recently co-authored with Rupert Sheldrake and Terence McKenna, *The Evolutionary Mind: Conversations on Science, Imagination & Spirit*, published 15 Jan 2015. Introduced to LSD by one of his students in 1967 when he was Professor of Mathematics at Princeton University in the USA, he stated in one published article:

> There is no doubt that the psychedelic revolution in the 1960s had a profound effect on the history of computers and computer graphics, and of mathematics, especially the birth of postmodern maths such as chaos theory and fractal geometry. This I witnessed personally.

Carl Sagan

Professor of astronomy at Cornell University for many years, Sagan and his works received numerous awards and honours, including the NASA Distinguished Public Service Medal; the Pulitzer Prize for General Non-Fiction; and the Hugo Award. He exemplifies the connection between mind-expanding drugs and scientific brilliance, for it is accepted within the scientific community's 'psychedelic circles' that this renowned astronomer, astrophysicist and cosmologist ingested LSD. In 'Psychedelics Encyclopaedia', written by the respected psychedelic historian Peter Stafford, he is listed as one of many famous people who ingested this substance. Though he never openly spoke about this fact, an essay in his book *Broca's Brain*, titled *"The Amniotic Universe,"* reviews Stanislav Grof's extensive and revolutionary LSD research. Sagan's use of words strongly suggests he is speaking from personal experience since he demonstrates a deep and perceptive familiarity with the effects of LSD, MDMA, DMT and Ketamine. Also the emphasis of his discussion is on the effects of LSD in particular, speculating that: *"the Hindu mystical experience"* of union with the universe *"is pre-wired into us, requiring only 200 micrograms of LSD to be made manifest."*

Andrew Weil,

Andrew Weil M.D., is an internationally recognized expert on 'integrative medicine', which combines the best therapies of conventional and alternative medicine. Several of his books have become New York Times bestsellers and he has appeared on the cover of Time Magazine twice, in 1997 and 2005. The New York Times recently wrote "Dr Weil has arguably become America's best-known doctor." Long interested in the medical potential of psychedelics, he was asked, when delivering a lecture at the April 2010 MAPS Conference in San Jose California, how psychedelics have influenced his perspective on medicine, and what sort of therapeutic potential he thought they had. His reply was:

> I think they've been a very profound influence…they made me very much aware, first of all, of the profound influence of consciousness on health…if they were legally available I think that I would use them as teaching tools to show people that you can change chronic patterns of illness, because even if you aren't cured of an illness the psychedelic may show you that it's possible…

Daniel Ellsberg

Political activist and former United States military analyst, Daniel Ellsberg became an icon after he made important military information public. While employed by the RAND Corporation in 1971, he released to The New York Times and other newspapers 'Pentagon Papers', a top-secret Pentagon study of U.S. government decision-making in relation to the Vietnam War. This 'act of conscience' helped turn public opinion against the Vietnam War, and contributed to the demise of President Richard Nixon. Along with charges of theft and conspiracy, Ellsberg was charged under the Espionage Act of 1917 - accusations carrying a total maximum sentence of 115 years imprisonment. However, due to governmental misconduct and illegal evidence gathering, combined with a solid defense presented by Leonard Boudin and Harvard Law School professor Charles Nesson, Judge Byrne dismissed all charges against Ellsberg on May 11, 1973. Ellsberg was later awarded the Right Livelihood Award in 2006.

He is also known for having formulated an important example in decision theory, the Ellsberg paradox. Ellsberg admitted taking LSD on a couple of occasions in the early 1960's and it seems reasonable to speculate that there is a significant possibility that this might have influenced his act of conscience nearly ten years later.

John Cunningham Lilly

Neuroscientist scientific pioneer and considered by many to be the most important figure in the field of electronic brain stimulation – the first person to map pain and pleasure pathways in the brain. He also pioneered an entire branch of science exploring interspecies communication between humans, dolphins and whales, and invented the world's first sensory deprivation chamber, a device that has been steadily growing in popularity over the past three decades. During his psychedelic research of the early 1960's, Lilly was one of the early LSD pioneers, using it to chart the inner landscapes of the human brain, inside his self-developed isolation tank. Within those dark, still waters, Lilly ingested huge doses of acid and delved deep into his mind in an attempt to imprint and re-program his mental circuits toward enlightenment and self-realization. However unfortunately, it would appear that for a few years - until he wisely chose to stop using it – his unwise, excessive use of the drug known as Ketamine, resulted in a significant disturbance of his mental balance, causing him to hallucinate that aliens were in constant contact with him, giving him important messages about the planet.

Bill Wilson (Alcoholics Anonymous)

One fact that might shock or astonish some readers, is that the co-founder of Alcoholics Anonymous (AA) believed LSD could be used to cure alcoholics, and he credited the drug with providing him with spiritual experiences that helped him to recover from debilitating depression. *"More and more it appears to me that the experience has done a sustained good,"* he wrote on 4th December 1956. *"My reactions to things totally, and in particular, have very definitely improved for no other reason that I can see."* In a 1957 letter to the science writer and philosopher Gerald Heard, Wilson wrote: *"I find myself with a heightened colour perception and an appreciation of beauty almost destroyed by my years of depressions…I am certain that the LSD experiment has helped me very much ".*

It was August 1956, approximately 20 years after setting up the Ohio-based sobriety movement, that Wilson took his first LSD trip, at the Veterans Administration (VA) hospital in Los Angeles. This was supervised by Betty Eisner, an American psychologist known for pioneering the use of LSD and other psychedelic drugs as adjuncts to psychotherapy, and by Sidney Cohen, a psychiatrist in Los Angeles. Based on his own experiences with LSD, Wilson was convinced that the substance could help *"cynical"* treatment-resistant alcoholics achieve a *"spiritual awakening"* that would put them on the path to recovery.

Betty Eisner wrote down Wilson's thoughts and intentions at the time: *"Alcoholics Anonymous was actually considering using LSD,"* Eisner recorded. *"Alcoholics get to a point in the programme where they need a spiritual experience but not all of them are able to have one."* According to the anonymous author of his official biography, Wilson felt LSD *"helped him eliminate many barriers erected by the self, or ego, that stand in the way of one's direct experiences of the cosmos and of god"* and he *"thought he might have found something that could make a big difference to the lives of many who still suffered"*.

Although it was Wilson's goal to include LSD treatment within the Alcoholics Anonymous program, most members of the AA organization were fiercely opposed to it, and since LSD was made illegal a few years later Wilson never had any chance of introducing the substance into the AA 12 step program. However, Wilson was *"so intrigued by the spiritual potential of LSD"* he formed an experimental group that included Father Ed Dowling, a Catholic priest and Eugene Exman, Harper's religious book editor.

Oscar Janiger

Oscar Janiger was a Los Angeles psychiatrist in the 1950s who was interested in testing the therapeutic effects of LSD on consenting patients. He received his own complimentary private supply of the drug from Sandoz, the manufacturers, in exchange for an agreement to document patients' experiences. Vanity Fair Magazine wrote that his experiments dominated his practice due to the increasing popularity of the treatment within Hollywood Circles. Assisted by Dr. Sidney Cohen, Janiger expanded his efforts into a "creativity" research study through U.C.L.A., where writers, painters, and musicians such as André Previn experimented with the drug.

Aldous Huxley became one of the first in Los Angeles to take LSD, soon to be joined by many others, including the writer Anaïs Nin. The screenwriter, Charles Brackett, asserted that on LSD he experienced *"infinitely more pleasure"* from music, and the director Sidney Lumet, supervised by former chief of psychiatry for the U.S. Navy, experienced three *"wonderful,"* sessions. The most notable, being one in which he relived his birth, and after relating the experience to his father, he discovered the 'experience' was factually accurate and not mere illusion.

Indeed, time after time in interviews, former patients recounted how it changed their perception of the universe and their place in it. Most agreed with Sidney Lumet, who says LSD provided *"remarkable revelations"* that he continues to consider very useful to this day.

Famous Authors, Actors, Actresses and Artists who used LSD

Rupert Sheldrake - Cambridge biochemistry don, Harvard scholar and fellow of Clare College. Author, public speaker.

I was interested in altered states of consciousness, so I tried lsd. It revealed to me regions of the mind that no one had taught me about in my neurophysiology classes. I felt there was a huge gulf between the scientific explanation — the nerve impulses, the ions across cell membranes, the mechanisms — and the actual experience of expanded consciousness. It made me wonder if I could achieve the same awareness without drugs. That's when I started meditating.

Oliver Wolf Sacks – Author, Professor of neurology and psychiatry at Columbia University

I think hallucinogens made me more open to some of my patients' experiences...I'm glad I had the experience. It taught me what the mind is capable of.

Eckhart Tolle - Spiritual teacher and author of bestseller, The Power of Now

I'm not recommending this but for some people it can give them a first glimpse of what it means not to be burdened by continuous mental commentaries. But it doesn't really raise your consciousness, it simply amplifies sense perceptions...Everything was vibrating, there was intensity of smell, hearing, the visual, tasting, everything was amplified…some people say "wow, the world can be so alive". It always is, you just don't know it because of the screen of your thinking.

Colin Wilson - English Existentialist philosopher and author

The effects of mescalin or LSD can be, in some respects, far more satisfying than those of alcohol. To begin with, they last longer; they also leave behind no hangover, and leave the mental faculties clear and unimpaired. They stimulate the faculties and produce the ideal ground for a peak experience.

Susan Blackmore - English freelance writer, lecturer, author of The Meme Machine

The ultimate psychedelic, whose discoverer is fit and well at a hundred years old, is LSD…Not only can it induce mystical experiences, but can treat neurosis and alleviate pain and fear in the terminally ill. We may be wasting a potential "wonder drug".

Walter Houston Clark - Professor of Psychology of Religion, Author

The psychedelic drugs are simply an auxiliary which, used carefully within a religious structure, may assist in mediating an experience which, aside from the presence of the drug, cannot be distinguished psychologically from mysticism. Studies have indicated that, when the experience is interpreted transcendentally or religiously, chances are improved for the rehabilitation of hopeless alcoholics and hardened criminals.

Michel Foucault - French philosopher, author social theorist, literary critic.

In 1975 he took LSD at Zabriskie Point in Death Valley National Park, later calling it the best experience of his life. "an unforgettable evening on LSD, in carefully prepared doses, in the desert night, with delicious music, nice people, and some chartreuse."

Richard Alpert ("Ram Dass) – Spiritual teacher, Former Professor of Psychology at Harvard

I didn't have one whiff of God until I took psychedelics.

My friends from Silicon Valley all used acid, and they took what they learned from psychedelics into technology. The creation of personal computers and the Internet was inspired in part by psychedelics.

Stephen John Fry - English comedian, actor, writer, presenter.

LSD reveals the whatness of things, their quiddity, their essence. The wateriness of water is suddenly revealed to you, the carpetness of carpets, the woodness of wood, the yellowness of yellow, the fingernailness of fingernails, the allness of all, the nothingness of all, the allness of nothing.

Robert Greene - American author of five international bestsellers:

I did a lot of psychedelics. I went to Berkeley in mid-70s. Before that I was doing LSD in high school. It was the era. My favorite was peyote. It's the greatest. It's unbelievable. I was heavily into Carlos Castaneda, I don't know if he's still popular now, the Don Juan stories which I thought were amazing. There's a lot of mescaline and peyote in those...I feel like that opened my mind to something. I have no regrets...I think it can be a very creative tool, it can open up your mind. It can be dangerous if you go too far.

Robin Skynner - Eminent British Psychiatrist and Co-author with John Cleese of Families and How to Survive Them

During that first experience through LSD...I seemed to lose all my own defences and need for self-deception, so that I could see my own faults clearly and accept myself despite them too. This seems to be a common experience — many similar ones were reported by the great psychologist William James in his book The Varieties of Religious Experience...For me it was like seeing a wonderful distant land from the top of a mountain. You knew that no matter how many more times you went up the mountain to look at it again, you still wouldn't really get any closer to what you'd seen. To get to it you had to go back down and make your way along the ground, which I've been attempting to do ever since. So I'm enormously grateful for that glimpse the drug gave me of what was possible.

Abraham Harold Maslow - Eminent American psychologist best known for creating "Maslow's hierarchy of needs".

In the last few years it has become quite clear that certain drugs called "psychedelics," especially LSD and psilocybin, give us some possibility of control in this realm of peak-experiences. It looks as if these drugs often produce peak-experiences in the right people under the right circumstances, so that perhaps we needn't wait for them to occur by good fortune. Perhaps we can actually produce a private personal peak-experience under observation and whenever we wish under religious or non-religious circumstances. We may then be able to study in its moment of birth the experience of illumination or revelation. Even more important, it may be that these drugs, and perhaps also hypnosis, could be used to produce a peak-experience, with core-religious revelation, in non-peakers, thus bridging the chasm between these two separated halves of mankind.

Tom Robbins - American author named one of the 100 Best Writers of the 20th Century by Writer's Digest magazine

Frankly, the day I ingested 300 micrograms of pure Sandoz LSD was the most rewarding day of my life, the one day that I would not trade for any other...On that fateful day, I experienced in a direct, first-hand, concrete and thoroughly rational way that 1) time really is relative, 2) every daisy in the field has an identity just as strong as my own and 3) what we smugly mistake for solid form in our "realistic" world is actually some strange fluid dance of molecular wonder. How could knowledge like that, lucidly demonstrated, fail to alter a person's life?... They enhanced my life -- psychedelics can enhance the life of any intelligent, courageous person, and they might even represent our last great hope for planetary survival -- but they didn't replace my life or become its central focus...The psychedelic drug doesn't exist that can make a creative genius out of a hack or turn a neurotic weenie into a happy fully conscious human being. You have to bring something to the table. And be willing to risk your belief systems.

Robert Anton Wilson - American author of 35 influential books

Now imagine these gigabytes of information entering your brain not in two years, but in two nanoseconds...Like English poet William Blake we have found "infinity in a grain of sand" and the deeper we look, the deeper the abyss grows...LSD seems to suspend the imprinted and conditioned brain circuits that normally control perception/emotion/thought, allowing a flood - an ocean - of new information to break through. The experience will seem either very frightening or exhilaratingly educational, depending on how rigidly you previously believed your current map contained "all" the universe. Since I learned that no model equals the totality of experience long before I tried LSD, I never had a bad trip; but I have seen enough anxiety attacks and downright wig-outs in cases of the naive and dogmatic that I have never favoured or advocated LSD's promiscuous use by the general population. As J.R. "Bob Dobbs says, "You know how dumb the average citizen is? Well, mathematically, by definition, half of them are even dumber than that...While splashing about and trying not to drown in this ocean of new information, you generally experience a second LSD surprise: an explosion of newfound energy within your own body...usually followed by something loosely called "near-death experience" or "out of body experience…In my case, after a few years I found myself seemingly forced to choose between mysticism and agnosticism. I solved that problem, for myself anyway, by choosing agnostic mysticism in the tradition of Lao-tse: "Something unknown, unspeakable,/ before Earth or sky,/ before life or death,/ I do not know what to call it /So I call it Dao"

Sam Harris - American author, philosopher, neuroscientist

At age 19, he and a college friend tried MDMA, better known as ecstasy, and the experience altered his view of the role that love could play in the world.

I realized that it was possible to be a human being who wished others well all the time, reflexively….This is not to say that everyone should take psychedelics. As I will make clear below, these drugs pose certain dangers…It has been many years since I took psychedelics myself, and my abstinence is born of a healthy respect for the risks involved. However, there was a period in my early twenties when I found psilocybin and LSD to be indispensable tools, and some of the most important hours of my life were spent under their influence. Without them, I might never have discovered that there was an inner landscape of mind worth exploring…The positive experiences were more sublime than I could ever have imagined or than I can now faithfully recall. These chemicals disclose layers of beauty that art is powerless to capture and for which the beauty of nature itself is a mere simulacrum. It is one thing to be awestruck by the sight of a giant redwood and amazed at the details of its history and underlying biology. It is quite another to spend an apparent eternity in egoless communion with it. Positive psychedelic experiences often reveal how wondrously at ease in the universe a human being can be—and for most of us, normal waking consciousness does not offer so much as a glimmer of those deeper possibilities…However, as the peaks are high, the valleys are deep. My "bad trips" were, without question, the most harrowing hours I have ever endured, and they make the notion of hell—as a metaphor if not an actual destination—seem perfectly apt. If nothing else, these excruciating experiences can become a source of compassion. I think it may be impossible to imagine what it is like to suffer from mental illness without having briefly touched its shores.

Douglas Rushkoff - American media theorist, writer, columnist, lecturer, graphic novelist

For me, the most illuminating thing about psychedelics was the insight that I had been living in a particular reality tunnel that had been constructed for me and that I constructed for myself, and we all kind of live in these reality tunnels, and there's ways to remove some of the filters and some of the constructs temporarily in order to see, or at least see second-hand through the chemical, that there's a whole bunch of other ways of looking at things. It set me on a mission, really, since college, when I had those experiences, to help people get that the reality we're living is much more "up for grabs" than most of us acknowledge on a daily basis. To use the programming metaphor, that reality is open source, and that if you learn the codes through which it's programmed, you can be a reality programmer rather than just a user. And that we walk around our daily lives mistaking a lot of what is actually software, for hardware. That there's stuff we accept as given circumstances, as the way things are, that are actually the way things happen to be. And many of them are the way things happen to be because other people decided that's the way they should be.

Gordon Sumner (also known as "Sting") - English musician and actor.

His comments on the Shamanic Psychedelic Ayahuasca:

> I may be out of my gourd, but I seem to be perceiving the world on a molecular level, where the normal barriers that separate "me" from everything else have been removed, as if every leaf, every blade of grass, every nodding flower is reaching out, every insect calling to me, every star in the clear sky sending a direct beam of light to the top of my head. This sensation of connectedness is overwhelming. It's like floating in a buoyant limitless ocean of feeling that I can't really begin to describe unless I evoke the word love…Before this experience I would have used the word to separate what I love from everything I don't love…Now all is swamped in this tidal wave of energy which grounds the skies to the earth so that every particle of matter in and around me is vibrant with significance. Everything around me seems in a state of grace and eternal.

Susan Sarandon

The Academy and BAFTA Award winning actress Susan Sarandon, whose successful career has spanned decades, is known for her political and social activism for a variety of liberal causes. She became a UNICEF Goodwill Ambassador in 1999, receiving the Action Against Hunger Humanitarian Award in 2006. She also makes no secret about the fact that she very much respects the profound, deeply moving, mind-expanding effects of psychedelics, having ingested the Amazonian sacramental psychedelic Ayahuasca a number of times, alongside psilocybin mushrooms.

I've done ayahuasca and I've done mushrooms and things like that…
But I like those drugs in the outdoors—I'm not a city-tripper… I like
doing it in the Grand Canyon, or in the woods. You want to be prepared and not have responsibilities. It does remind you of your space
in the universe—your place in the universe—and reframe things for
you. I think you can have some very profound experiences.

Frances McDormand

The award-winning actress Frances McDormand is one of the few
performers who has achieved the Triple Crown of Acting. In 1997,
she won the Academy Award for Best Actress for Fargo; in 2011 she
won the Tony Award for Best Actress in a Play for the original Broad-
way production of Good People; and in 2015 she won the Primetime
Emmy Award for 'Outstanding Lead Actress in a Miniseries'. In one
interview she admitted: *"I really, really enjoyed LSD, and I really enjoyed mushrooms very much… We needed a PR person for that LSD! It
was very profound. Very profound."*

Larry Hagman

The Actor Larry Hagman, famed for his role as the Texan Oil Magnate J.R. Ewing, in the soap opera *Dallas*, wrote of LSD in his au-
tobiography: "more than anything else, the experience changed
my way of looking at life and death." In an interview with MAPS
founder Rick Doblin he exclaimed:

LSD was such a profound experience in my life that it changed
my pattern of life and my way of thinking… We're so infinitesimal
in the whole scheme, in the universe. If you look out there and
you see hundreds of billions and trillions of stars with systems as

big as our whole Milky Way, it's just infinite, I guess. Could there be a finite end? I think that death and LSD go hand and glove. If you have a large chance of having an enlightening, life-enhancing experience, or making death easier for you, even enjoyable and something to look forward to, what's wrong with that?

Huston Smith

Huston Smith was appointed professor and chair of the philosophy department at MIT from 1958 to 1973. While there, he participated in experiments with psychedelics that professors Timothy Leary and Richard Alpert (aka Ram Dass) conducted at Harvard University. He then moved to Syracuse University, where he was Thomas J. Watson Professor of Religion and Distinguished Adjunct Professor of Philosophy, until his retirement in 1983 and current 'Emeritus' status. His book *The World's Religions* (originally titled *The Religions of Man*) has sold over two million copies and remains a popular introduction to comparative religion.

- For those who think that psychedelics are illusory spiritual experiences, this video of Huston smith will confirm the authenticity of these experiences: https://www.youtube.com/watch?v=0ifvuzdO3uY

Alan Watts

- The renowned philosopher/theologist describes his views and experience on LSD: https://www.youtube.com/watch?v=g-A3C8FEscw

William James

Sometimes labelled "The Father of American Psychology", Author William James was an American philosopher and psychologist and trained physician. He was one of the leading thinkers of the late nineteenth century and is believed by many to be one of the most influential philosophers the United States has ever produced.

Although LSD was discovered after his death, he is included in this section because he experienced a state of consciousness - induced by Nitrous Oxide - that is very reminiscent of LSD experiences:

One conclusion was forced upon my mind at that time, and my impression of its truth has ever since remained unshaken. It is that our normal waking consciousness, rational consciousness as we call it, is but one special type of consciousness, whilst all about it, parted from it by the filmiest of screens, there lie potential forms of consciousness entirely different.

Ken Kesey

Following the success in 1962 of his novel One Flew over the Cuckoo's Nest, writer Ken Kesey embarked on a cross-country bus trip in 1964 with a bunch of friends, ingesting copious amounts of LSD. The book by Tom Wolfe 'The Electric Kool-Aid Acid Test' chronicled their experiences.

> I got high on psychedelics before I was ever drunk. I never smoked. Then LSD came by. And to me it was the most wonderful thing that had ever happened...And I don't know of anybody who hasn't come back from that being more humane, more thoughtful, more understanding.

Alex Grey

Best known for his depictions of the human body that "x-ray" the multiple layers of reality, revealing the complex integration of body, mind, and spirit and the body's meridians and chakras. Grey's unique series of 21 life-sized paintings, the Sacred Mirrors, present the physical and subtle anatomy of humanity in the context of cosmic, biological and technological evolution. A mid-career retrospective of Grey's works were exhibited at the Museum of Contemporary Art, San Diego in 1999.

His paintings have been featured in *Newsweek Magazine* and on *Discovery Channel*. His books include *Sacred Mirrors: The Visionary Art of Alex Grey*, his philosophical text, *The Mission of Art*, and *Transfigurations*. Sounds True released *The Visionary Artist*, an audiotape of Grey's art, philosophy and vision practices.

Grey openly acknowledges that he fuels his creative expression with LSD experiences. He claims that one particular trip in 1976 changed the entire course of his life:

> Twenty-five years ago I took my first dose of LSD. The experience was so rich and profound, coupled as it was with the meeting of my future wife, Allyson, that there seemed nothing more important than this revelation of infinite love and unity. Being an artist, I felt that this was the only subject worthy of my time and attention. Spiritual and visionary consciousness assumed primary importance as the focal point of my life and art. My creative process was transformed by my experience with entheogens.

Cary Grant and Betsy Drake

Cary Grant is a legendary leading actor of classic Hollywood, considered to be the American Film Institute's second greatest male star of all time. He was one of the first within the acting world to experience and recognize the value of the therapeutic application of LSD, after being introduced to it by his third wife, Betsy Drake, in the 1950's before it was outlawed. In an attempt to deal with her failing marriage and troubled childhood years, Betsy underwent weekly sessions of LSD therapy for several months. She credits her LSD therapy with *"giving me the courage to leave my husband"* and for the first time to truly speak her mind.

> After an LSD session, one morning in bed while we were both having breakfast, Cary asked me a question and I said, 'Go fuck yourself.' He jumped out of bed…and slammed the bathroom door. That was the true beginning of the end.

She and Cary ended their 13 year-long marriage in 1962, but remained friends for the rest of his life. LSD intensified Betsy's interest in the mental-health field and she began studying at U.C.LA's Neuropsychiatric Institute, later enrolling at Harvard, where she earnt her Masters of Education in psychology, specializing in psychodrama therapy where patients act out problems instead of discussing them. Significantly, when interviewed 50 years later in her London home, the radiant smile accompanying her enthusiastic comments about LSD, make it clear that Betsy's optimism about the drug has still not waned. Her memories of her experiences under LSD are still crystal-clear, and the revelations still vivid:

> The unconscious is like a vast ocean. You don't know where you are going to go. There is no past, present, and future—all time is now. The

amazing thing about the drug is the things you see. The palm trees look different. Everything looks different, and it teaches you so much.

Cary Grant's enthusiasm for the treatment is perhaps best encapsulated by a comment he once made about LSD: *"Oh those wasted years, why didn't I do this sooner?"* He underwent around 100 sessions of LSD therapy at a high-end California clinic, which he claims brought him *"inner peace"* which he failed to achieve through yoga, hypnotism and mysticism. *"I know that, all my life, I've been going around in a fog. You're just a bunch of molecules until you know who you are."* In *Look Magazine's* 1959 issue *"The Curious Story Behind the New Cary Grant,"* he spoke of his LSD therapy, saying:

> …at last, I am close to happiness…I wanted to rid myself of all my hypocrisies. I wanted to work through the events of my childhood, my relationship with my parents and my former wives. I did not want to spend years in analysis…I learned many things in the quiet of that small room. I learned to accept the responsibility for my own actions and to blame myself and no one else for circumstances of my own creating. I learned that no one else was keeping me unhappy but me; that I could whip myself better than any other guy in the joint.

Grant claimed LSD deepened his sense of compassion for people, his understanding of himself, and helped cure his shyness and anxiety in social situations. One of the drug's greatest pre-illegality proponents, Grant gave interviews to various women's magazines on its transformative effects, encouraged friends and subsequent wives to take it. However, on one occasion Grant's enthusiasm got the better of him when his fourth wife, Dyan Cannon, claimed that prior to their divorce he had attempted to *"force-feed"* her LSD, believing that it would transform her into the *"shiny new wife who could effortlessly meld as one with her husband"*. Until his death, Grant remained a strong advocate for LSD and other psychedelic substances.

Clare Boothe Luce

Inspired by the work of the earlier-mentioned psychiatrist Oscar Janiger, playwright and former American ambassador to Italy, Clare Boothe Luce, was so impressed with her experiences on LSD that she in turn persuaded her husband, Time Magazine publisher Henry Luce, to try the psychedelic. He subsequently wrote and published some very positive articles about the drug's potential in his magazine in the late 50s and early 60s, praising Sandoz and LSD itself as providing *"an invaluable weapon to psychiatrists."*

The following represent an interesting range of discussions of the psychedelic experience:

https://www.youtube.com/watch?v=FqAZ_7nBHS8

www.youtube.com/watch?v=jPLimDG_HVY

https://www.youtube.com/watch?v=zrYl9krZksk

https://www.youtube.com/watch?v=GMjtAu1JqOg

https://www.youtube.com/watch?v=LTcLHNPcL2w

https://www.youtube.com/watch?v=MxvQusr9cwc

Chapter Two

Dr Berceli's Trauma Release Exercise Method

Michael's attempt to articulate a concise summary of the TRE process is quite admirable. He maintains a factually accurate description of TRE, covering the most salient components of this physical approach to relieving stress, tension and trauma symptoms, while including the theoretical and practical foundations upon which TRE is based.

Dr David Berceli

Dr Berceli's method for dealing with trauma is entirely different from traditional approaches which are often fundamentally cognitive-based. Instead of attempting only to change thought patterns and emotional responses to bring about beneficial changes in the psyche, Berceli asserts that an important additional resource for resolving traumatic issues lies in treating the body directly, and his technique, which reduces discussion and analysis of a person's problems to a minimum, can be used effectively in conjunction with formal psychotherapy.

In his many years of working with traumatised clients, he has constantly observed that trauma-induced behaviour is exceptionally difficult to treat solely with the use of traditional crisis intervention techniques that depend fundamentally upon cognitive processing. This is due to a variety of psychological, neurological and physiological reasons. Primarily it is important to remember that trauma behaviour is often an illogical, instinctual response not under the control of the rational mind. In other words, when faced with real pressures of trauma or extreme stress, we can't merely *think* or *talk* our way out of it.

But evolution has provided us with an in-built neuro-biological mechanism that helps to dissolve severe stress patterns arising from sudden or prolonged psychologically disturbing situations, or traumatic life experiences, because, as Berceli explains:

> As a human species, we are neurologically, biologically and physiologically designed to experience, endure, survive and even evolve from traumatic events. We are genetically coded to let go of and recover from trauma as a way of ridding ourselves of any experience that obstructs or interferes with the natural evolutionary process of the human body. Trauma is often a process for growth, change and evolution into a stronger disposition.

However, although this genetically encoded natural process has proven itself to be highly effective, our cultural training generally overlooks body-based methods, but fortunately, Dr Berceli has provided us with the means to rapidly awaken this currently dormant mechanism.

When a potentially traumatizing situation occurs, which is an event that is perceived as a dangerous threat to one's existence – (the threat may be a genuine physical danger, or merely emotional, psychological or even imaginary in origin) - the most primitive parts of the brain – the limbic system and brainstem – take over. The body then responds by mobilizing primal defence mechanisms in readiness for self-defence via the fight, flight, and freeze responses, which are designed to protect us from this perceived threat. This is when the muscles powerfully contract to protect us from harm and massive amounts of cortisol create a resistance to pain combined with a life-threatening sense of urgency that motivates action to escape harm. Simultaneously, adrenalin intensifies energy and alertness, enabling peak performance that is further enhanced by blood, oxygen and glucose being diverted to the muscles, to maximize physical prowess, and to the sensory and motor cortex of the brain, sharpening sensory awareness and enhancing reflexes.

These physiological responses are usually accompanied by anger, aggression or fear, and the totality of all these physical and emotional responses enhance our capacity to survive. However, in the aftermath of potentially traumatizing situations, if these same survival responses are not efficiently discharged as nature intended, the experience becomes emotionally and physiologically overwhelming, often for extended periods of time that can last years or even an entire lifetime.

This condition, known as 'Post Traumatic Stress Disorder' (PTSD), reflects a serious malfunctioning of a biological system designed to alert us to, and help us cope with real danger. This malfunctioning is analogous to a faulty smoke alarm whose siren continues long after the smoke has cleared and the threat has gone. So the state of an individual suffering from PTSD who is constantly in the 'emergency mode', is analogous to a person who is continually responding to a faulty smoke alarm siren by mobilizing their fight or flight response as though there is a real fire happening.

This is because instead of the pent-up energy being released immediately following the traumatic situation, the body stores it in its muscles and connective tissues. The deep physical contractions and permanently raised levels of cortisol and adrenalin constantly feed negative thoughts, feelings and images, associated with the traumatic event. The emotional and rational parts of the brain convert the suffering this creates into intense emotions such as hatred, rage, distrust, or shame, or into a negative ideology of existence, or worse, a desire for revenge. All of this, nourishes and reinforces the unresolved trauma with all its symptoms.

> Traumatic symptoms are not caused by the 'triggering' event itself. They stem from the frozen residue of energy that has not been resolved and discharged; this residue remains trapped in the nervous system where it can wreak havoc on our bodies and spirits. (*Waking the Tiger*, Peter A. Levine, PhD).

In a futile attempt to discharge this blocked energy and the accompanying negative emotions, the brain unconsciously attempts to recreate the trauma. This is done either by reproducing situations similar to it, or by using memory to 'reanimate' the traumatizing scenario. This serves to bring it back into the present moment so that it can be re-lived and re-experienced – an act that can be a 'vicious circle' of self-imprisonment. According to Berceli, in the case of PTSD, aroused energy generated at the time of the event, which is prevented from being discharged, remains trapped in a bio-neural-physiological loop that causes a repetition-compulsion pattern of behaviour.

> Unfortunately, this tactic of 'replaying' the traumatic scenario again and again is not only entirely ineffective, but it usually intensifies the symptoms of trauma, thereby increasing feelings of anger and depression. And then, as Berceli points out, trauma becomes, "*an overwhelming and seemingly unbearable life experience.*"

No wonder, says Berceli, that victims of unresolved trauma often become perpetrators of violence and abuse either toward themselves or toward those closest to them. A common example of this 'replaying process' is seen in the case of abused children who choose to enter into abusive relationships as adults. For when exposure to trauma has been long-standing (as it is for children with histories of child-hood physical or sexual abuse), a person may develop certain endur-ing behaviour patterns. These include difficulty in trusting others, irregular moods, impulsive behaviour, shame, decreased self-es-teem, irritability and anger, or depression, and this is likely to exert a profoundly negative effect on long-term intimate relationships, as partners suffer the' fallout' from the unresolved stress and trauma.

Dr David Berceli has become an internationally renowned trauma-tologist, since the launching - around ten years ago - of his unique, revolutionary method that helps to heal trauma. For 15 years he lived and worked in war-torn countries in Africa and the Middle East, and has provided specialized trauma recovery assistance to U.S. military personnel, national and international relief agencies, and govern-ment and non-government organizations whose staff are living and working in trauma-inducing environments. To date, he has conduct-ed his trauma relief training in more than 30 countries worldwide.

His training has been used successfully in large military popula-tions, as well as in large traumatized civilian populations exposed to natural or war-related disasters. The method is especially appro-priate since it is essentially non-verbal and thus easy to demonstrate and teach, which makes it applicable in cultures where the 'victims' might not speak the same language as the therapist.

Berceli's approach was inspired by his observation of animals in the wild. Animal researchers have noted that the physiological response of tremoring, innate to all primates and mammals, provides crea-tures in the wild with an in-built immunity to stress. This enables them to return to normal life after a highly charged life-threatening experience, (even if this involves a loss of members of the flock) - without developing any PTSD symptoms whatsoever.

This cathartic process can be observed in the violent involuntary shaking and spontaneous deep breathing of gazelles in their natural habitat, as they discharge intense biochemical energy when they have found safety after escaping death from a lion attack. It is also seen in the tremors passing through the body of a horse after a fall, in the wing flapping of ducks after a fight, and in the rapid trembling of a frightened guinea pig or rabbit.

Berceli realized that this trembling is nature's physiological mechanism for discharging energy and releasing contractions in the muscles and connective tissues of the body once an emergency has ended, and the hyper-aroused fight or flight or freeze response is no longer required. The parasympathetic nervous system then takes over to restore relaxation and equilibrium in the body-mind which can now recover and repair any damage caused by the traumatic event.

To illustrate how this same mechanism is supposed to function in human beings, Berceli likes to present to the participants of his courses an ideal example of this biological de-traumatizing process, by showing a video of a bear who ran from danger. After escaping, the bear lay on his back, trembling uncontrollably. The bear then let out a huge, loud sigh, calmed down and continued with his normal activities seemingly as if nothing had happened.

This is what allows wild animals to survive without living in constant fear or panic, under conditions that would deeply traumatize most humans and keep them in a constant state of hyper arousal. Animals are free of this dysfunctional state as their natural uninhibited tremoring always occurs whenever they experience potentially traumatic events, thereby instantly allowing them to release stresses and tensions so that they can rapidly heal and build increased resiliency to cope with future traumas.

Although humans are similarly designed to rebound equally rapidly from traumatic circumstances, mostly, we tend to use our mind's ability to override this natural, cathartic discharge. We do this through rationalizations and judgments that are rooted in the traditional cultural perception of trembling as being a pathological expression of stress; a diagnostic characteristic of panic attacks, social phobias and generalized anxiety disorder that is associated with a reduced ability to cope.

This gross misunderstanding, combined with the intrinsic need that most people have to 'be in control' and not show any sign of weakness or vulnerability, has caused the vast majority of humans to suppress and deaden this natural shaking mechanism instead of allowing it to organically restore the body to balance under conditions of severe stress. And the more 'control-oriented' a person is, the more difficult it is for them to allow these trauma-releasing tremors to emerge when needed.

Berceli's incredibly simple, yet effective system is based upon six easy-to-learn movements, called "Trauma Release Exercises" (TRE). These exercises invoke the crucially important primordial neuromuscular reflex within our bodies that gives rise to entirely involuntary mild to vigorous trembling and shaking. These rapid intermittent muscular contractions, scientifically known as 'neurogenic tremors', gradually release deep chronic muscular contractions from the core muscles of the body – the psoas muscles, which play the most active role in the fight/flight/freeze response, the paraspinal muscles (small muscles attached to the vertebrae parallel to the spine that help maintain alignment) and the abdomen.

This group of muscles comprise the nucleus and source of most somatic (body) tension triggered by stress or trauma. When the contractions in this area are released, this simultaneously returns the autonomic nervous system to a state of balance, lowering cortisol and adrenalin to normal levels, which allows for the gradual dissipation of the anxiety, depression or anger that was fuelled by the earlier state of constant hyperarousal.

It has been used extensively with US military personnel so they can modulate their physical/emotional responses during deployment. A key advantage of this system in a military context is that it does not have to be facilitated by a counsellor, since soldiers can rapidly be trained to facilitate one another. This tends to neutralize in most cases, a resistance to undergoing therapy which is typical of many soldiers suffering from PTSD.

The TRE technique requires some preliminary movements which stress and stretch the leg and calf muscles until muscle fatigue creates some trembling. The person is then required to lie on their back allowing the tremors to begin activating in the pelvis and lower back. Following repeat sessions over a period of several days or sometimes weeks, the tremors eventually spread through the body, until they are distinctly felt along the entire spinal column from the sacrum to the cranium, as well as in the shoulders, arms and legs.

After around 15 minutes of shaking, there often arises an incredible sense of release and freedom from chronic physical contractions; negative thought patterns and painful emotions dissolve. In addition, feelings of helplessness, anger and depression are replaced by a sense of empowerment that is accompanied by clarity of mind that restores mental and emotional equilibrium and renewed direction in life.

What makes this technique so special, distinguishing it from all other approaches, is that because the shaking is involuntary, the individual is not obliged to use (and should not use), any conscious effort to control their body or mind. This is unlike most other relaxation/

meditative techniques which rely upon the practitioner's active participation.

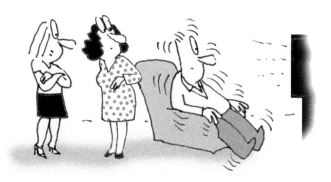

"It's his Trauma Release exercise. After the news he'll be doing it on the floor."

This is because TRE operates primarily through the unconscious part of the mind, so theoretically speaking, if one wishes, one could actually watch TV, or listen to music, and allow the shaking to do all the work, without paying any attention to it.

For some people, allowing the mind to be distracted by another activity enables the body to release tension more effectively. This is because the 'distraction' tends to prevent the ego and other cognitive or emotional activity from interfering in the natural process, since thinking and analysing can inhibit and override the body's ability to 'let go'. For many people however, the process of focusing on the body, and on the arising emotions, can contribute to the healing. In the end, each individual must work out what works best for them.

Another attractive feature of TRE is that it can be used safely and successfully by both young and old, regardless of age, race, gender, religious affiliation, or economic status and can be self-taught through a short instructional video or two-hour workshop.

Since it is generally experienced as relaxing or pleasurable, and has almost immediate effects in reducing hyper-arousal, very little motivation is required to develop a daily practice and this is why it is an excellent adjunct to many other body-based techniques such as yoga, tai chi and meditation which have also proven to be very effective in reducing stress. However the latter usually require extended practice to yield their effects, whereas in TRE, beneficial effects are often reported in the first or second session.

It is helpful if one understands in advance the difference between the different types of shaking which can occur. Sometimes the shaking can be very vigorous, and the movements very visible, indicating that the large muscles in the body are breaking up massive 'iceberg-like' stresses and tensions. This type of shaking tends to continue until these large blockages dissolve, thereby liberating energy to flow more easily. At this point, finer shakes/tremors, often take over, and these sometimes diminish to just a gentle vibration.

These smaller tremors serve to dissolve the less obvious and deeper forms of tension that we are constantly holding, and during any particular session the tremors may ebb and flow with greatly varying intensity, or even stop altogether for a while. All one needs to do is trust that the body is doing exactly what it needs to do at any particular moment, because according to Berceli, tremoring is an individual process and there is no right or wrong way. This is because the body understands what it must do to soften and relax the patterns of tension, conflict and trauma that have accumulated over the years. So at any given moment our body releases what it needs to release and therefore, to judge sessions as 'good' or 'bad' can impede their natural flow and reduce efficacy.

While some people experience significant emotional release during the process, others may experience no emotional response whatsoever. Some may experience intense memories of a trauma, while others may have no memory or recollection at all and experience only the physical shaking while still achieving a significant physiological and psychological release. All responses are sufficient because each session is unique and provides precisely what is needed at the time.

One should always remember that there is no 'goal' since the objective is just to 'let it be' and allow whatever happens to emerge naturally. However, it is not unusual, as a result of the phenomenon known as 'muscle memory', for there to be a profound discharge of intense emotions that have been 'frozen' into the muscle tissue, and which re-surface as a result of the intense shaking which liberates these congested emotions from the connective tissue and muscles. This discharge may derive from the awakening of recent traumas, as well as from old feelings that may have been forgotten for decades.

This can potentially have an especially benevolent cathartic effect on the entire body-mind, rapidly dissolving the symptoms of even the most unpleasant traumas. However, if one begins to feel emotionally overwhelmed, uncomfortable, or frightened, and there is a desire to stop the procedure, then one should do so immediately. One should never allow strong emotional reactions to continue for more than a few minutes during any given session, unless one is supervised by an experienced TRE practitioner. To end the procedure, the only requirement is to straighten the legs and lock the knees for a few minutes while remaining in the lying position until one feels grounded again in the present moment.

You know you are doing TRE in the right way when you feel you are shaking from a place of safety and can tolerate and control your emotions, thoughts, feelings, and sensations independently of external supervision or regulation - David Berceli calls this 'self-regulation'.

If you are not already at this stage then it is always advisable to have a TRE practitioner, or perhaps friends or family sit with you until this state of self-regulation is active. As mentioned earlier, it highly recommended to use this technique in adjunct with various forms of psychotherapy that specialize in treating trauma, especially when the emotions and memories associated with past trauma are particularly intense. In such instances discussion and analysis are often essential.

If you are doing TRE for the first time, it is recommended that you only tremor for a maximum of 15 minutes every other day. Once you have been doing TRE for a few weeks, you can lengthen your tremor time and/or increase your frequency at your own discretion.

Eventually, it is ideal to use TRE on a daily basis to release any negative emotions and physical tensions caused by work stress, excessive worry, conflict in relationships, and it is also extremely effective at reducing pain and speeding up recovery arising from overtraining or injury.

In many cases, all that will be required to learn the method for home use is one single supervised session by a trained TRE practitioner.

Some readers however may prefer to learn the technique entirely on their own, using David Berceli's book on the subject: *Revolutionary Trauma Release Process: Transcend Your Toughest Times*. For those wishing to learn the technique and also read case histories: *Shake It Off Naturally: Reduce Stress, Anxiety, and Tension with (TRE)*

- Anyone interested in trying out this trauma release exercise system should visit Berceli's two websites: where they can find information about his charity and a list of practitioners who teach the procedure.

www.traumaprevention.com

http://www.bercelifoundation.org/s/1340/aff_2_home.aspx

- Excellent example of TRE doing what it is supposed to do:

  https://www.youtube.com/watch?v=NbbaFTTvxU0

CHAPTER THREE

CANINE DIAGNOSTICS

E veryone knows that dogs are highly intelligent creatures with a multitude of potential skills. They lead the blind, detect the whereabouts of people lost in forests, mountains, or buried under avalanches and collapsed buildings, and they can find the tiniest traces of explosives. In the past decade they have astounded even the most sceptical of scientists by demonstrating that they can surpass cutting edge diagnostic technology in their ability to detect certain illnesses simply by sniffing them out; this incredible ability often results in life-saving diagnoses for afflictions that otherwise would often remain undetected until it is too late.

The idea that some maladies have a characteristic odour goes back millennia. In the time of Hippocrates, around 400 BCE, it was reportedly common for patients to cough and spit on hot coals to generate a smell that the physician would sniff to ascertain the disease. But it has taken humans thousands of years to recognize the amazing potential that canines have for this type of diagnosis.

In 1989, dermatologists Williams and Pembroke, at London's King's College Hospital, wrote in The Lancet (a revered medical journal founded in 1823) about a woman, whose dog persisted in smelling a particular mole on her leg, on one occasion even trying to bite the lesion off. Although previously this woman had not been in the slightest bit concerned, prompted by her dog, she sought medical advice. The mole was excised and histology tests revealed it to be an extremely early-stage malignant melanoma measuring just 1.86 millimetres in thickness. Since that time, the woman has remained well and there has been no sign of recurrence.

A second Lancet letter, published in 2001, reports the case of a 66-year-old male who developed a rough patch of skin on the outer side of his left thigh, which over a period of 18 years had grown slowly to about 1-2 centimetres in diameter. Causing occasional itching whenever it became dry and scabby, it had been diagnosed as eczema and treated, unsuccessfully, with various topical agents, including anti-fungal and steroids. A pet Labrador, Parker, that had been living with the man for a couple of years, suddenly began pushing his nose against the man's trouser leg - sniffing at the lesion beneath it - which prompted him to consult his family physician. In September 2000 the lesion was cut out, and an examination revealed it to

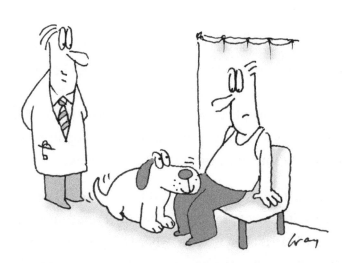

Don't mind Prince - he's just trying to tell you that you have cancer.

be a basal cell carcinoma. Following this, his dog showed no further interest in the area.

Having seen Williams' and Pembroke's report, Cognetta, a dermatologist in Florida USA, teamed up with a retired police-dog handler who had served in Vietnam leading the K9 bomb unit. Using conventional sniffer-dog techniques, they trained George, a Schnauzer, to recognize in vitro malignant melanoma samples, and then introduced him to a patient with several moles that had all been diagnosed as cancer-free. However, one particular mole caused George to go crazy with excitement, and subsequent excision of the lesion confirmed very early-stage malignant disease.

"This is how it (medical detection dogs) started…it was all anecdotal", Dr John Church told the inaugural international conference on medical bio detection, in Cambridge, UK, in September 2015. Dr Church, a retired orthopaedic surgeon, is the founder of the International Biotherapy Society, and he has played a pivotal role in the advancement of the field of medical dog detection.

These dogs are trained to detect minute odour traces created by diseases, and are currently employed in research into the fight against cancer. They can also help to improve the safety and quality of life, of people with incurable, life-threatening diseases such as diabetes and epilepsy, when they are trained as *"Medical Alert Assistance dogs"* to detect minute changes in blood sugar levels and other hormone related odour changes that precede impending medical events. They will then either signal their owner to take remedial action, or get help from others if their owner is incapacitated - in some cases they will even fetch vital medical supplies.

The dogs have proved to be invaluable carers for diabetics with "brittle" Type 1 diabetes, a form of the illness which is not preceded by the typical warning signs of headaches, sweating, dizziness or extreme tiredness. This means the sufferer can feel perfectly fine one moment, and then suddenly, without any warning, undergo a seizure. Medical alert assistance dogs are trained to watch over individuals with this problem, and are known as *"Hypo Alert Dogs"*, since they immediately notice the instant their owner begins to become hypoglycaemic (low blood glucose level). They are trained to respond in a number of ways – by alerting their owner, by fetching a blood glucose testing kit or by pressing a specially installed alarm in their owner's home.

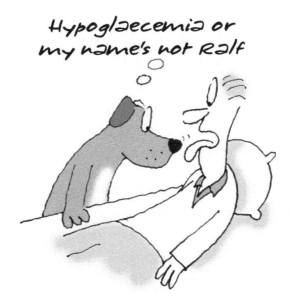

"Polo", a black Labrador, is one of numerous dogs trained by the charity called *"Medical Detection Dogs"* (discussed later in this chapter) to detect pending attacks caused by this type of diabetes. Each night, Polo, sleeps beside 12 year old Gemma Faulkner's bed to keep an eye and a 'nose' on her because Gemma, who has "brittle" type 1 diabetes, sometimes experiences dangerously rapid alterations in her blood sugar levels, which can put her into a coma even while she sleeps. "Polo" can smell specific changes in Gemma's body odour which signal the moment these changes begin to occur. Whenever he detects this, he'll grab his toy bone and push it into her sleeping parents' faces to alert them. Gemma was diagnosed with brittle type 1 diabetes just before she was 3 years old. She could never sense her blood sugar level dropping and thus never woke up when she was having night-time hypos, which obliged her parents to test her for hypoglycaemia night and day around 15 times per 24 hour stretch.

Other medical detection dogs have been trained to assist people who are afflicted with Addison's disease, by warning them of impending attacks that could lead to collapse and unconsciousness, which enables the sufferer to take immediate and effective pre-emptive remedial action to prevent such a crisis. Life-saving 'Nut Allergy Dogs' have prevented those with a severe allergy to nuts (normally peanuts), from enduring potentially fatal anaphylactic shock. These dogs will warn their owner, whenever they are about to consume foods containing nuts such as peanuts, or peanut oil, which is hidden in so many foods, but easily sniffed out by these dogs.

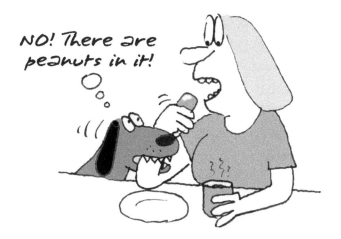

The Medical Detection Dog charity also provides canines to take care of victims of epilepsy. More than half a million people in the UK suffer from this illness and around 30% of them can't control it through medication, and live constantly with the worry that an epileptic episode may happen at any time. These 'seizure alert' dogs can warn their owner up to 50 minutes before an oncoming attack, providing them with sufficient time to find a place of safety and privacy while they have their seizure. Thanks to these trained canines, epileptics can safely attend to their daily tasks like shopping, having a bath, or cooking, free of the fear that they might suddenly be overwhelmed by an unexpected attack of epilepsy, which could put them in danger.

The biology behind this canine ability to detect various illnesses is fascinating. All smells, ranging from the pleasant aroma of freshly cut grass, to the odour of pungent cheese, are produced by molecules of the substance that is causing the smell, diffusing in the air. These molecules are detected by scent (olfactory) receptors in the nose which send signals to the brain which then interprets the smell.

Scientific studies have demonstrated that even in the earliest stages of cancer – long before it can be detected by any current imaging modalities or blood testing technology - that malignant cancer cells are already producing volatile organic compounds. These are exhaled on the breath and excreted in the urine (and maybe also through the skin's sweat glands), and although the odour of these compounds is well below the threshold of the human olfactory sense, the same does not apply to dogs, as they possess a sense of smell infinitely stronger than ours.

The percentage of a dog's brain devoted to analysing odours is around 50 times larger than that of a human, so whereas humans have around 5 million olfactory (smell) receptors/neurons, the dog has approximately 300 million, and in addition, at the rear of their nose, they have a second smelling device - that we don't possess - called Jacobson's Organ. This 'double' smelling system explains why trained dogs can easily detect cancer's unique odours. Alexandra Horowitz in her book *Inside of a Dog*, explains the consequence of this difference in more concrete terms: *"We might notice if our coffee's been sweetened with a teaspoon of sugar; a dog can detect a teaspoon of sugar in a million gallons of water: two Olympic sized pools full."*

Although anecdotal evidence of the existence of "canine diagnosticians" has existed for decades, it was not until 2004 that the first clinically rigorous investigation of cancer detection by canines was reported by Carolyn Willis and colleagues (*British Medical Journal* 2004). During this study, dogs were trained by individuals working for the earlier mentioned charity "Medical Detection Dogs", to detect the "odour fingerprint" for bladder cancer, by smelling urine samples from patients and healthy controls. Six dogs of varying breeds were used, none of which had been trained for previous scent work. Overall diagnostic accuracy was 41%, with the best dog achieving 56% (compared with the 14% success rate expected from chance alone). However, Italian research in the *Journal of Urology*, conducted by the *Department of Urology* at the *Humanitas Clinical and Research Centre* in Milan, far surpassed these results:

Two female German shepherd dogs were successfully trained to detect prostate cancer in the urine, simply by sniffing for gassy compounds, which are specific to prostate cancer. They sniffed the urine of 900 men - 360 with prostate cancer and 540 without. One dog was successful at identifying prostate cancer in 98.7 per cent of cases, while the other dog achieved 97.6 per cent accuracy.

These results are especially significant, given the fact that prostate cancer is the most common cancer in men in the UK, with more than 40,000 cases diagnosed every year. The most common test for detecting prostate cancer, the PSA blood test, has proved to be unreliable, since it gives a false positive in 3 out of 5 cases, requiring 75% of men to undergo further invasive tests.

Readers who, after reading this chapter, now feel inspired either to purchase a medical detection dog or to contribute to the aforementioned charity that trains them, can locate this incredible organization at the following address: www.medicaldetectiondogs.org.uk

They are without doubt the true pioneers in this field, at the leading edge of this humanitarian medical approach, and importantly, they are running the first NHS ethically approved proof-of-principle trial, exploring the ability of dogs to detect breast cancer. This has attracted the interest of many reputable members of the medical profession, who are also interested in canine potential for detecting other cancers such as lung and colorectal cancers. 'Medical Detection Dogs' also intend in the future, to assist with research into the development of electronic systems ('E' noses) that hopefully will provide cheap, non-invasive tests for the early detection of a wide variety of cancers.

But buyers beware! Do not waste your time trying to find a 'better deal' by purchasing 'medically' trained dogs from other companies offering the same service, unless they have been verified as authentic by the aforementioned charitable organization. There has already been one case example of an unscrupulous business, claiming to provide trained medical dogs, when in fact they were just ripping off their customers. "Service Dogs Europe (SDE)" sold 'assistance' dogs, with severely inadequate training, for the seemingly 'bargain' price of €8,000. And to make things worse, many of the dogs were ill – with hip dysplasia being a common problem. Their trainers were expected on average to train from scratch around 16 of these dogs each month. Fortunately an employee of this company blew the whistle on them and they were closed down very rapidly.

Founded in 2008, the Co-Founder and Chief Executive and Director of Operations of Medical Detection Dogs (MDD), Dr Claire Guest, was the director in 2003, of the first programme in the world to train dogs to identify cancer by odour. The findings of this study were published in the British Medical Journal in September 2004. Claire is the recipient of the "British Citizen Award" for 'life-saving work in the management of long-term illnesses and research into early cancer detection', and in May 2015 she was awarded a fellowship from *The Royal Society of Medicine.*

But it is her pet dog who is perhaps the real star of the show: The fox red Labrador, Daisy, detected Claire's breast cancer six years ago when Claire was 45, *"She kept staring at me and lunging into my chest. It led me to find a lump,"* Claire remembers. The tumour was deep in her breast. Her doctors said that by the time she would have discovered it herself, the cancer would have been very advanced: *"Had it not been drawn to my attention by Daisy, I'm told my prognosis would have been very poor".* Daisy was eventually awarded the *"Blue Cross Medal"* for her pioneering work in the field of cancer detection, where she has sniffed over 6,500 samples and detected over 550 cases of cancer.

Prince Charles' wife Camilla, Duchess of Cornwall, is patron of this charity. Betsy Duncan Smith, wife of the former Conservative Party leader, Iain Duncan Smith, is a trustee, and the charity has appointed the wildlife and science TV presenter Kate Humble as their Ambassador. Kate said: *"I was utterly blown away by my day at Medical Detection Dogs. The work they do is extraordinary."*

During question time at the House of Lords, Tory peer and Former Defence Minister, Lord Astor of Hever, raised the issue of using such dogs as part of the NHS:

> Each day that we sit in this House, we trust dogs' acute sense of smell of explosives to ensure our safety," the Tory peer said. "Research shows dogs detect human disease earlier than existing tests and this could increase survival rates and save the NHS millions of pounds.

Liberal Democrat Baroness Ludford called for more access to detection dogs for people suffering from diabetes, and Lord Prior responded favourably to her suggestion:

> The costs of training a dog is some £11,200 - considerably less than the cost of training a doctor, and I might add…The use of dogs to sniff urine is more accurate than conventional forms of detecting cancer.

Shadow Health Minister Lord Hunt said: *"That is a clear hint of the Government's new approach to the shortage of doctors."*

- Readers can watch an interview of with Dr Claire Guest on the following videos:

  http://www.bbc.co.uk/news/health-33834153

  http://www.nbcnews.com/nightly-news/video/these-dogs-are-using-their-noses-to-sniff-out-prostate-cancer-520407107854

- Watch Jade, a Labrador, in action taking care of making sure her owner with diabetes gives himself insulin when it's needed:

  http://www.itv.com/news/granada/update/2015-12-20/wonder-dog-jade-saves-owners-life-hundreds-of-times/

CHAPTER FOUR

EPLEY OMNIAX VERTIGO THERAPY

A lthough vertigo (dizziness) is a condition that affects all ages, the probability of being afflicted by it significantly increases as we get older. Though very rare in the under 35's, by the age of 75, 25% of North Americans and Europeans will have a balance disorder, and falls have become the leading cause of death among people over 65. Ninety million Americans go to health care providers because of vertigo, dizziness or balance problems.

Symptoms can range from a light feeling of nausea and/or a feeling of being off-balance, to a sensation that parallels being on a violent merry-go-round, where the surrounding world is spinning so fast that everything becomes a complete blur and one cannot possibly remain standing.

Vertigo can be a symptom of many different illnesses and serious disorders, but many types of vertigo, though not life-threatening, remain unresolved, and sufferers are told they just have to live with the disability together with all the lifestyle restrictions that go with it.

The Epley Omniax Chair may look like an amusement-park ride, but it's actually a sophisticated, $250,000 tool employed in the diagnosis and treatment of vertigo and other vestibular (inner ear) balance disorders. The machine derives its name from the inventor, Dr John Epley, an ear surgeon from Portland, Oregon, who achieved international acclaim in the early 1990's, after developing a technique called *'The Canalith Repositioning Procedure'*. It is now popularly known as *"The Epley Manoeuvre"* - a hands-on treatment that can be easily carried out by doctors and therapists, to treat many types of Benign Paroxysmal Positional Vertigo (BPPV).

BPPV is probably the most common cause of vertigo in the United States, characterized by brief recurrent episodes, often so disturbing that sufferers cannot work or carry out their daily activities. This form of vertigo was first described in 1921 by the Austro-Hungarian otologist, Robert Barany, who received the 1914 Nobel Prize in Physiology or Medicine for his work on the physiology and pathology of the vestibular apparatus.

It has been estimated that at least 20% of patients who present to the physician with vertigo, have BPPV. However, because BPPV is frequently misdiagnosed, this figure may not be completely accurate and is probably an underestimation.

Eventually however, Dr Epley saw numerous limitations to the aforementioned manual manoeuvre, and prior to his retirement, encouraged by his daughter, he developed the vastly superior technological alternative. Cathy Epley named the business which produces and sells the *Omniax System, 'Vesticon'* and from 2003 – 2006 she managed to gain around $3.5 million USD of grants to hire top engineers and technicians to develop the Omniax chair. Eventually, after stringent clinical trials testing its safety and efficacy, it achieved sales approval and clearance by the FDA in 2007.

Epley's Computerized Chair, with unique, patented diagnostic software, moves vertigo patients gyroscopically, in order to shift them into specific positions that enable the doctor to test each part of the inner ear, in order to determine the particular type of vertigo that is causing the problem. Currently, it is the only available clinical tool that offers comprehensive management – and frequently a permanent cure - for positional vertigo, caused by non-particle disorders, and for classic *Benign Paroxysmal Positional Vertigo* with its many variants. Often the treatment is completed in five to ten minutes, and most patients feel better immediately afterwards.

Inside the ear are three tiny canals that help us recognize the position of our body in space so that we can maintain balance. These canals are filled with fluid, and attached to the walls of the canal are tiny hairs that connect to nerve endings. The way the fluid washes against the hairs changes when your body is in different positions. When the fluid moves the hairs, nerve signals are sent to the brain. Those signals get translated in a way that lets you know what position your body is in.

BPPV occurs when tiny calcium carbonate crystals (canaliths) form in the inner ear and become dislodged. Floating freely, if the crystals bang around the canals, touching the hairs, it causes the sensitive nerve endings to send conflicting signals to the brain which create a false sensation of body movement, or the illusion that the surrounding environment is spinning around the body. If you have BPPV, the symptoms can be triggered by any sudden head movements, such as when you get up from lying down, roll over in bed, look up or down, or bend down. This sets these free-floating crystals in motion, causing these bouts of nausea and/or extreme dizziness which continue until the crystals settle down again.

It is very easy to diagnose BPPV, because accompanying the sensation is a characteristic flickering eye movement called nystagmus, which occurs as a result of what is known as the vestibulo-ocular reflex. Normally, when the inner ear tells your brain your head is moving, the brain then sends signals to the eyes to keep them focused. However, if the inner ear sends the wrong signals, as in BPPV, the brain tells the eyes to spin in an attempt to keep you looking ahead, and it is this which causes them to flicker.

How the Epley Omniax functions

Depending on the client's health history and symptoms, the specialist will determine if they are a suitable candidate for the Omniax. If they are, they will be seated in the Omniax chair, and safety belts and pads will be fastened across the shoulders, waist and legs to keep them safely secured and prevent them from shifting as the Omniax turns. A headrest positions the head appropriately to provide comfort and safety. This allows the operator to safely and precisely achieve any patient position, enabling a much wider range of treatment options than the *"Epley Manoeuvre"*. The latter is often not an ideal or safe option in the case of anxious, frail, or physically limited patients who suffer from bad neck or back problems or painful, stiff joints.

Because the chair rotates in all directions, allowing for 360° positioning in any plane, sometimes the client may be upside down, so users are requested to wear shorts or trousers.

When a person is "dizzy," their eyes jump or move back and forth, creating the previously mentioned phenomenon called "nystagmus. The client wears special infrared, night-vision goggles equipped with tiny video cameras, that relay the pattern of these eye movements directly to the computer which records them. Because the video cameras in the goggles are high resolution, they provide a crystal clear view of nystagmus, which reveals not only overt nystagmus motions, but also subtle, latent or transient nystagmus.

The client will not be able to see out of the goggles so that the vestibular system is obliged to attempt to control their balance without input from the faculty of vision. If the client's eyes move abnormally without visual input, this provides important clues to the type of vertigo afflicting them.

As the chair gyroscopes, the computer registers the precise body positions which trigger the nystagmus (which is invariably accompanied by feelings of vertigo) as well as the speed and pattern of these eye movements that are specific to each of the 'trigger' positions. The computer software provides, via independent analysis of each semi-circular canal throughout their 360° range, a clear differentiation between BPPV and other causes of position-related vertigo, which can arise from a variety of disorders in the ear as well as in the brain or elsewhere.

The resulting information, combined with knowledge of the precise positions which bring on the symptoms of vertigo, enables the doctor to program the chair for appropriate treatment. This is either from a menu of standard protocols or they can choose to develop their own customized/personalized 'freestyle manoeuvers' for each canal and condition.

If the cause is BBPV, the computer discloses the particular type that is causing the problem, as well as the exact location in the semi-circular ear canals of the errant calcium carbonate crystals that are responsible for the vertigo. The particular type of BPPV a person has, determines the procedures and positions that, with the assistance of gravity, will cause the calcium crystals to move out of the area where they are causing the vertigo, to the region of the inner ear – the vestibule – where they do not cause any further symptoms, and once there, these crystals automatically dissolve or are reabsorbed by bodily fluids in the ear.

This procedure of shifting the crystals out of the ear canals can be likened to the actions of guiding a ball through a puzzle maze to find the hole it is supposed to drop through. If the problem is straightforward, for example if the crystals located in the client's ear are in just one canal rather than in several canals, and moving freely instead of being trapped in one position due to the anatomy of the canal, and if that canal is one of the easier canals to navigate; then, just as a very simple ball maze requires only a few easy motions to complete the task, the treatment in the Omniax chair will also be simple. In such cases, one treatment will often be sufficient, and will consist of just a few simple manoeuvres to

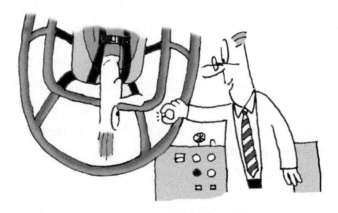

Here's the culprit. The little devil that's been causing your vertigo

tilt and roll the patient in a sequence of moves that steer the offending particles through the maze of the ear canals to a spot where the debris will no longer interfere with the balance, or cause dizziness.

More complex cases – as with more complex ball mazes - require multiple and more elaborate manoeuvres as well as more time, and the client may need to return for several repeat sessions. In the latter instance, the Epley Omniax allows the operator to monitor progress and review previous sessions using printed reports, session logs and customized video playback. In the end, the chair not only removes the cause of most types of BBPV, but the treatment is usually long-lasting and sometimes there is no recurrence.

Statistical analysis of controlled trials using the Omniax chair, have demonstrated that it can treat successfully more than 90% of BBPV sufferers, though approximately 50 percent of these patients will experience another bout and need further treatment after a lapse of around three years.

- The following is a two minute long YouTube video which concisely demonstrates the Epley Omniax chair in use:
  https://www.youtube.com/watch?v=cA3W35RlZYQ

- Video showing the Epley Omniax treating war veterans with traumatic brain injuries:
  https://www.youtube.com/watch?v=YRGgvY93Wdg

- The Epley Omniax Company video - medical practitioners explaining their findings:
  https://www.youtube.com/watch?v=Lioyscurh_w

- NBC news on 79 year old male vertigo sufferer undergoing Omniax chair treatment:
  https://www.youtube.com/watch?v=cfCcKGT2-WM

- News Coverage of an Audiologist in Florida demonstrating the Epley Omniax:
https://www.youtube.com/watch?v=Jwg_4mSzY2A

- Melbourne, Australia Royal Victorian Eye and Ear Hospital and the Epley Omniax:
https://vimeo.com/110958866

The Epley Manoeuvre (The Canalith Repositioning Procedure)

Access to the Omniax treatment outside the USA is extremely limited. The Omniax system is available in Australia and China, but at the time this chapter was written, it appears that in Europe, The vestibular unit at Rigshospital's ENT department in Denmark is the first and possibly the only hospital in Europe which currently offers testing and treatment on the Omniax Chair, and there is a waiting period of several months to get an appointment.

Vertigo sufferers who are prepared to wait this long for an appointment can find details at the following web address:

- https://www.rigshospitalet.dk/english/departments/centre-of-head-and-orthopaedics/department-of-otorhinolaryngology-head-and-neck-surgery-and-audiology/conditions-and-treatments/Sider/dizziness.aspx

BBPV sufferers in urgent need of treatment should try the very best alternative to the Omniax chair, which is the earlier mentioned Canalith Repositioning Procedure, popularly called 'The Epley Manoeuvre', (Canalith is the medical term for calcium carbonate crystals).

When John Epley developed this technique as a treatment for BBPV in 1980, he initially faced extreme scepticism, even derision, from his colleagues. *"Everyone thought it was crazy,"* Epley said. At the October 1980 meeting in Anaheim, California, where he introduced his idea, few believed Epley's claim to have developed an incredibly simple, extremely low-cost almost instant cure for the most common cause of chronic vertigo which afflicted thousands with crippling attacks of dizziness and nausea accompanied by involuntary twitches of the eyes that were triggered by just a casual tilt or turn of the head.

And these periodic attacks often tormented sufferers for years, baffling physicians whose only offer of treatment was medication, or - as a drastic last resort - surgical destruction of nerves to the inner ear, which impaired the patient's general balance and sometimes also their hearing.

Epley's Manoeuvre arose out of his experiments with plastic tubing that he and a colleague had shaped into a model of the inner ear. To simulate the free-floating errant calcium carbonate particles in the inner ear, that he believed were responsible for the vertigo attacks, he put BB airgun balls in the coiled tubes of the plastic inner ear model. Epley and his colleague then spent time playing with their construction, flipping and turning the hand sized model as one might a kid's puzzle, to work out a sequence of moves to reposition the tiny metal balls in other areas of the plastic inner ear. They hypothesized that if these BB airgun balls had been real-life calcium crystals in a human ear, that their manoeuvres would have rendered the offending particles harmless.

They began testing the moves they had developed on their patients, tilting and rolling them on an exam bench, imitating the successful moves they had made on their model ear. After they had successfully cured a number of vertigo sufferers using this approach, including one patient who had endured continual dizziness for more than a decade, they realized they'd hit upon a marvellous set of therapeutic manoeuvres that could revolutionize vertigo treatment by healing lifelong sufferers of this potentially life-destroying condition.

In 1992, he submitted a report to the journal of the American Academy of Otolaryngology. In it, he described the 100 percent cure rate of his "canalith repositioning" manoeuvre in 30 patients with almost 90 percent of his patients being cured by a single treatment.

The journal published the report and Epley's revolutionary method was finally recognized as a treatment for BPPV. Scepticism towards his discovery still continued among many in the medical profession, until 2001 when a review article in the prestigious New England Journal of Medicine, credited John Epley as the inventor of the *"treatment currently recommended for positional vertigo"* as the standard treatment for BPPV. One study revealed that, on average, patients spent more than $2,000 USD in tests and failed treatments, before being successfully treated with the Epley manoeuver or related procedures.

Amazingly, given the effectiveness of the technique, it was not until 2009 that the *American Academy of Neurology* recommended *The Canalith Repositioning Procedure* as the fastest, easiest way to cure BPPV. This was far superior to traditional treatments which have ranged widely from sedatives, to nerve surgery, to nothing at all. They asserted that unfortunately most patients who are likely to benefit from CRP may not be receiving it.

Dr.Terry D. Fife, an assistant professor of clinical neurology at the University of Arizona explains:

Instead of telling patients to 'wait it out' or having them take drugs, which can help with the nausea and vomiting, but not the underlying cause, instead, we can perform a safe and quick treatment that is immediate and effective.

He further explains that the technique is not taught in medical schools and most general practice doctors may have heard only rumours of this procedure as a quick, easy way to treat vertigo:

BPPV is the most common cause of vertigo (others include migraine and viral inner ear infections) and can be very debilitating if left undiagnosed and untreated, which happens more often than we'd like, as surprisingly few people — including medics — have heard of it.

While most ear, nose and throat departments and some neurologists offer these treatments, there can be a long waiting list for referral to someone who can perform these 'particle repositioning' manoeuvres.

In the UK, Dr Peter West, consultant audiological physician, at the Queen Alexandra Hospital, in Portsmouth, has come to exactly the same conclusions as Dr Fife.

Peter West sees about six patients a week with BPPV. *"In 50 per cent of cases, BPPV will get better on its own — the crystals make their way back to the correct part of the ear, or dissolve, although this can take weeks or months,"* says Dr West. And many have been suffering for years with the distressing condition, which can be rapidly diagnosed and treated with almost immediate results using the Epley Manoeuvre.

Dr West explains, *"These manoeuvres are quick to perform and will eliminate symptoms in a single treatment in around 90 per cent of cases, but awareness of BPPV is still not as high as it should be among the medical profession."* This means thousands of people, mainly the elderly, go without treatment for the distressing condition because doctors are unaware of how to diagnose and treat it. West said medics spend too little time learning about the workings of the ear:

> They simply have no idea how the inner ear works. And they do not know they are ignorant about it. It is as bad as that. I saw one patient who had BPPV for over 30 years and her GP had told her there was nothing that could be done. And I have had four or five patients who have had this for 15 years or more and they have just been told that they have to learn to live with it. It is a very important condition in the elderly. Because if they fall and they hurt themselves they could end up in long-stay wards. I had one patient who had suffered from it every day for 24 years until she came to me for treatment. We resolved it within five minutes. Another 92-year-old had been housebound for a year after being told his dizziness was part of getting older and he would have to put up with it, but two weeks after I performed the Epley Manoeuvre on him, he was out at Royal Ascot.

The following videos demonstrate and teach this manoeuvre which is incredibly simple to learn but which should only be administered by a trained professional:

- Video demonstration – "Epley manoeuvre" (no sound) https://www.youtube.com/watch?v=pa6t-Bpg494

- American Academy of Neurology instructional video of Epley Manoeuvre:
https://www.youtube.com/watch?v=hq-IQWSrAtM

- Mayo Clinic Video discusses the Epley Manoeuvre:
https://www.youtube.com/watch?v=utVcWuhPj3s

- Excellent Epley Manoeuvre teaching video by Dr Christopher Chang:
  https://www.youtube.com/watch?v=9SLm76jQg3g

The ideal way for trained professionals to master the Epley Manoeuvre is to learn from someone who is proficient in the technique, or alternatively they can learn by watching the above instructional videos and practicing on a willing subject who is *not* a vertigo sufferer.

However, the following *abbreviation* of an NHS guide to the Manoeuvre has been included to give the layman a rough idea of how easy it would be to learn the procedure:

Approximate instructions for the Epley Manoeuvre:

All stages of the following instructions for administering the Epley Manoeuvre are undertaken slowly and smoothly, with the head and neck supported at all times.

- Start with patient sitting on couch. Turn patient's head toward affected side (e.g. the direction of movement which tends to trigger the vertigo).

- Pause in this position for 30 seconds and then lie the patient flat, while supporting head which remains turned to affected side. Pause in this position for 30 seconds.

- Keeping head looking in same direction but now ask patient to gently move to lie on hip and shoulder of good side. Then turn head toward good ear. Patient will now be looking at floor, with chin close to shoulder. Pause in this position for 30 seconds.

- Gently bring patient to sitting position. Ensure head position does not change relative to trunk (chin still on shoulder of good side). Pause for 30 seconds.

- Finally, turn head to centre and flex neck to put chin on chest in one movement. Pause for 30 seconds.

Caution: As should be obvious, this is only a *very rough guide* and should *not* be used on a patient, since this procedure needs to be carried out by a trained professional and with great care as if it is performed incorrectly it could be damaging, most especially if someone has neck or back problems or diseases such as osteoporosis.

Post-manoeuvre instructions.

Patient is requested not to drive home after an Epley treatment. Patient is to avoid lying flat for 2 nights after the treatment. For a further 5 nights, avoid lying on bad side: Sleep on good side with pillow behind back to act as a barrier to rolling over.

CHAPTER FIVE

HELMINTH THERAPY

Biotherapy refers to any medical practice involving the use of living creatures to aid in medical diagnosis or treatment.

Helminth Therapy, which requires the ingestion of 'helminths' to improve the functioning of the immune system, is a very recent, not yet accepted, medical approach which lies within the aforementioned field of Biotherapy.

Helminths (the word is derived from the Greek meaning "worms") are parasitic worms such as hookworms, whipworms, and threadworms that have evolved to live within a host organism on which they rely for nutrients. It seems clear that they have always plagued mankind, for the eggs of intestinal helminths have been discovered in the mummified faeces of humans dating back thousands of years. Many of the characteristic clinical features of helminth infestation can be recognized in the ancient writings of Egyptian medical papyri, Hippocrates, and the Bible.

Readers who, at this stage, are recoiling from, and are extremely sceptical towards the idea that a remedy using parasitic worms could ever become a validated, mainstream medical practice, should pay close attention to the following facts which may well convince them to change their viewpoint:

The medicinal application of Maggots and leeches are two classic examples of ancient biotherapies that have been used by physicians for thousands of years. These treatments, first described by Persian physicians in 980, and mentioned in 2500 year old Ayurvedic texts, also featured in the writings of the father of modern medicine, Hippocrates. In 2004 both maggots and leeches were approved for mainstream medical use by the Federal Regulators of the FDA, who classified them as the *"first live medical devices"*. Nowadays, any licensed physician in the U.S. and in the UK can prescribe maggot therapy, which utilizes live, disinfected maggots (fly larvae) for the purpose of cleaning out the necrotic (dead) tissue within a wound.

Increasingly employed to treat severe wounds such as surgical amputations, burns, diabetic ulcers, skin cancer and gangrene, there is also evidence that maggots reduce the risk of post-operative infections, and in 2011, worldwide, approximately 50,000 maggot treatments were applied to wounds.

Since 2004, leeches have been routinely used to drain blood from swollen faces, limbs and digits after reconstructive surgery. This is because their saliva contains a natural anticoagulant, Hirudin, which thins the blood and dilates the blood vessels to increase blood flow, facilitating the leeches ability to 'drink'. This anticoagulant simultaneously prevents and dissolves, congested or clotted blood, thereby reducing inflammation, and in addition the fresh, nutrient-rich oxygenated blood that reaches the area, speeds up the healing process.

Ken Dunn, consultant burns and plastic surgeon at the South Manchester Burns and Plastic Surgery Service said:

> We use leeches to establish a flow of blood through tissue where
> there is congestion of blood, usually because the flow of venous

blood out is not adequate...If this is not done the tissue will die from that congestion of blood.

Studies led by Andreas Michalsen, a researcher at the University of Duisburg-Essen in Germany, indicate that leech therapy may also be a useful means of reducing osteoarthritic pain and inflammation.

Readers interested in leech therapy can contact the following website for more information: www.guysandstthomas.nhs.uk/leaflets

Hopefully cynical readers will now be more open to the idea of Helminth Therapy, an experimental type of immunotherapy, which arose out of research into the role of certain parasites as "biological response modifiers" (BRM's).

BRM's are the active agents of immunotherapies. 'Activation immunotherapies' use BRM's in order to elicit or amplify the immune response, for instance, to reject and destroy dangerous bacteria or cancerous tumours. Whereas 'suppression immunotherapies' use BRM's to suppress or dampen an abnormal immune response, in order to treat 'autoimmune disease' such as multiple sclerosis, arthritis, and certain kinds of allergies that are the immunological equivalent of friendly fire; this occurs when the immune system becomes overactive and damages the body by reacting toward its own organs and/or tissues as though they were the 'enemy'.

Helminth "immunotherapy" involves the deliberate ingestion of controlled numbers of benign intestinal "helminths" (parasitic worms) or helminth ova's, which function as 'suppressant' BRM's. These calm down an overactive immune response, thereby alleviating the symptoms of a wide variety of chronic autoimmune disorders.

In answer to an obvious question: which worm works best for which illness? Researchers, suppliers and consumers have identified a few promising helminths that are most useful for targeting Crohn's disease, ulcerative colitis, inflammatory bowel disease (IBD), Celiac disease, multiple sclerosis, asthma and other allergies. Consequently, almost all helminth users ingest one of the following four different species - the rat tapeworm, pig whipworm, human whipworm, or human hookworm. The choice being determined by the particular worm that is best adapted to healing the specific ailment afflicting the person.

What is also highly significant about these four species of parasitic worms is that when supervised, none of them can cause serious health problems. This is because they don't reproduce in humans, and they are neither infectious nor contagious so they cannot spread from person to person. They also don't migrate within the body, and importantly, all of them can be very easily and rapidly eliminated with anti-worm medicines.

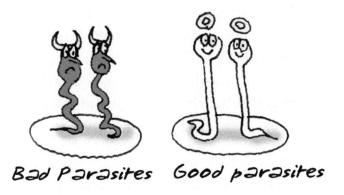

Bad Parasites   Good parasites

Although Helminth Therapy is not yet a legal mainstream medical practice, two particular helminths, Pig Whipworms and Hookworms, have already been approved for clinical research on human volunteers. These 'medical worms' have been granted licences as 'investigational medicinal products' (IMP) by the USA Food and Drug Administration and by the UK equivalent, Medicines and Healthcare Regulatory Authority.

Filmmaker Sharon Shattuck featured these critters in her documentary **Parasites: A User's Guide.** *"We all have a really negative opinion of parasites,"* Shattuck said from New York. *"It equates to everything evil in our society. Many worms are hazardous pathogens, but not all parasites are created equal."*

Shattuck profiled several success stories concerning individuals who claimed that their ingestion of 'benevolent' parasites had cured them from allergies that formerly had been so severe that they were unable to go outside. *"These are people at their wits' end,"* Shattuck said, *"But these worms are able to tap into the inflammatory response and turn it down. It acts as a soothing mechanism"*.

Helminth therapy was inspired by empirical evidence which reveals that in less developed countries south of the equator, where Helminthic infection is most widespread, there is a very low incidence of allergies and autoimmune diseases such as type 1 diabetes, ulcerative colitis, celiac disease, Crohn's disease and multiple sclerosis. This contrasts starkly with the incredibly high incidence of these same diseases in developed Western countries of the Northern Hemisphere, where Helminthic infection has virtually been wiped out. This difference is especially significant given the fact that the National Institute of Health estimates up to 23.5 million Americans suffer from autoimmune disease and that this statistic is rapidly rising.

Gastroenterologist Robert W. Summers, MD, of the University Of Iowa College Of Medicine explains:

It turns out that countries where inflammatory bowel disease (IBD) is common are those industrialized, developed nations like the U.S., where there are no intestinal helminths. Conversely, where helminths are prevalent, the incidence of IBD is very low... In fact, Crohn's and ulcerative colitis only really emerged in the U.S. during the 1920s and 1930s, when we began to shift to improved plumbing and sanitation and we no longer fertilized soil with both human and animal waste. Until then, these parasites were very common. And we didn't have much IBD.

And the increased rate in the incidence of these autoimmune diseases over the past 100 years is too short a period for the cause to be a result of genetic changes in humans.

As a result of these empirical observations, a growing number of scientists now support what is known as the *"Old Friends Hypothesis"*, first proposed in 2003 by Professor Graham Rook. Until about 150 years ago, nearly everyone who ever lived was probably infected with some type of parasitic worm. The Old Friends Hypothesis points out that public health improvements in the 20th century - due to the development of vaccines, effective medical care, environmental sanitation and the provision of clean drinking water - have diminished or eliminated the prevalence of many natural, benevolent microorganisms and parasites that are essential for an optimized immune system. This is because our immune system evolved with, was shaped by, and came to depend upon, the constant bodily presence of these creatures; especially certain parasitic worms which regulate our immune system, preventing it from going haywire.

What seems ironical about this situation, is that we are, quite rightly, extremely concerned with the biodiversity in the outside world, for instance, with matters such as saving the rainforest. Yet at the same time we utterly disregard the internal ecosystem of our body, thereby screwing up the biodiversity inside of us – or perhaps this is just another example of *"The Law of Correspondence"* which tells us that our outer world is nothing more than a reflection of our inner world – as within, so without.

Dr Joel Weinstock, chief of gastroenterology and hepatology at Tufts Medical Center in Boston, explains to Discovery News, *"Many of these worms are bio-engineered for humans. We adapt to them; they adapt to us. They become like an organ, just like your heart, your spleen or your liver."*

There are two fundamental types of immune responses: the "fight and kill" response, which causes inflammation and attacks foreign invaders, and the regulation response, which dampens down angry cells after their attack. But if the immune system becomes dysfunctional the regulation response can break down, because, says Weinstock. *"If something that gets in your body can be killed with a fly swatter, but your immune system decides to use the atomic bomb, that's not going to be very good for your lungs, skin or other organs,"* says Weinstock.

However, helminths can prevent our body from attacking itself, because our immune system has developed a symbiotic relation with these parasites: Helminths secrete/excrete molecules that stimulate the production of 'regulatory T cells'. These are anti-inflammatory immune cells which serve to suppress immune responses of other cells in order to reduce the intensity of inflammatory, as well as other immune responses. This is a biochemical tactic that developed to keep the human immune system from killing the helminths and simultaneously serves as a 'thermostat, that maintains our immune system's inflammatory response at a level that is neither too hot nor too cold, but just right, thereby preventing inappropriate immunological responses toward our own body or toward harmless antigens such as pollen, or dust, or cats, or benign food groups.

"People who host helminths can still mount an inflammatory attack on pathogens, but they don't set off self-destructive immune bombs against harmless substances or their own cells. Helminths don't make our immune system lazy or less effective—they make it smarter"," says William Parker, associate professor of surgery and an immunology researcher at Duke University Medical Center.

Interestingly, one of the first recorded success stories of Helminth Therapy dates back to the mid-1970's when John Turton, whilst working at the UK's Medical Research Council Laboratories in Surrey, intentionally infected himself with hookworms in an attempt to relieve his chronic hay fever. He hosted the parasites for two consecutive summers, and his allergy symptoms were banished, but returned when he eliminated the worms. (The Lancet, vol. 308, p 686).

A more recent pioneer of Helminth Therapy is Jasper Lawrence. As a child he was identified as 'gifted' but failed to fulfil his potential when he dropped out of his Oxbridge group in hard sciences, due to his dabbling in drugs. He explains:

> I used to suffer from awful asthma and allergies, to the extent that I could only breathe comfortably if using oral prednisone in such high doses that I developed lipomas and became for the first time in my life very obese. My aunt told me about a documentary she had seen on the BBC about the beneficial effects of worms on relieving asthma.

The story that most inspired Lawrence was the ongoing research of Professor David Pritchard, an immunologist at Nottingham University. While in the field in Papua New Guinea in the late 1980s,

Pritchard noted that patients infected with the *Necator Americanus Hookworm* were rarely subjected to the whole range of autoimmune-related illnesses, including hay fever and asthma.

To begin with, Lawrence tried to get accepted as a participant on one of the various studies investigating the helminth phenomenon. But when that and all his other efforts to obtain hookworm proved fruitless he relates, *"I went first to Cameroon and later to Belize to obtain hookworms."* Hookworm's infiltrate a new human host when larvae, hatched in human excrement, penetrate the soles of the feet, enter the bloodstream, travel through the heart and lungs and are swallowed when they are coughed up from the pharynx. In the tropics, left untreated, they can be deadly but, they are not infectious and in small numbers they are harmless, and very easily eradicated.

In Cameroon, Lawrence spent a couple of weeks travelling to remote villages, where he walked about barefoot in outside areas used specifically for defecation:

> The big fear was that I'd come back with the wrong disease, river blindness or elephantiasis, or Dengue fever, or whatever. On the other hand I had seen exactly how my life had declined in the last five years with asthma. Modern medicine seemed to have nothing to offer me except palliative drugs. So really, I felt there wasn't a choice for me.

Several months later, without any confirmation that he had been successfully infected by hookworm, he recalls, one day in the spring he was out driving, *"I had the window of my car rolled down,"* he says. *"Normally if I did that at the start of spring I would spend the rest of the day blowing snot, swollen red eyes, and the works. But it didn't happen."* And formerly Lawrence had been so allergic to cats that if he touched one and touched his face he would get a red mark. His eyes would swell shut. *"So I deliberately exposed myself to a cat... And nothing happened."*

Lawrence had experienced a total remission of his asthma and seasonal allergy symptoms. Inspired by his incredible recovery, in 2006 he cofounded an online worm therapy business *"Autoimmune Therapies,"* originally teaming up with Jorge A. Llamas, an alternative therapies doctor, and Garin Aglietti, another self-infected believer who had healed his psoriasis with hookworm. They had patients fly into southern California and cross into Mexico for treatment. But this partnership ended shortly after its inception, and Lawrence continued to sell worms solo in Santa Cruz. He explains:

> Since I founded Autoimmune Therapies in 2006 we have treated dozens of clients with a variety of diseases: allergies (food and airborne), multiple sclerosis, Sjogren's syndrome, psoriasis, ulcerative colitis, Crohn's disease, and autism. The results have been remarkable, far better than those possible using modern drugs.

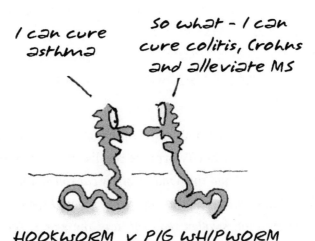

HOOKWORM v PIG WHIPWORM

After harvesting his hookworms which are plucked from his own faeces, Lawrence washes them repeatedly in various antimicrobials and antibiotics, prior to packaging them up in sterile liquid and then they are ready to go. Customers can choose between the options of swallowing a dose of whipworm, or applying a Band-Aide of hookworms which allows the worms to seep into the skin within several hours. The only side effects are minor itching, which can be relieved by using Benadryl.

The client should begin to notice improvements in their health one or two months after the initial infestation has taken place and Lawrence sells five years of this treatment, with extensive support services, for $3,900. A figure he justifies with the comparative cost of MS drugs for example, which might be closer to $150,000. However, although his website does not display prices, the cost must have dropped dramatically by now, or he would be out of business, since competing companies, such as www.wormswell.com currently sells batches of hookworms for just $200.

Spurred by online testimonials, Lawrence's business slowly grew for nearly three years until November of 2009, when the FDA visited Lawrence's home and ordered him to stop selling the worms, as they had recently been classified as an 'investigational new drug' that would only become legal pending successful clinical trials. Apparently, the FBI then paid him a visit after contacting PayPal and freezing his bank account, and they left at 5.30pm on a Friday, promising to return on the Monday. By 1am on Saturday - fearing retribution from the FDA - Lawrence and his girlfriend Michelle had already crossed the border on foot, into Mexico at Tijuana, where he knew there was no passport control. They eventually made it back to the UK where he continued to sell his worms via his online company www.autoimmunetherapies.com.

Although Lawrence continues to move around Britain he won't disclose his street address, but it seems clear that his substantial contribution to the field of Helminth Therapy has been acknowledged by doctors worldwide. He was invited to deliver a presentation to gathered scientists and doctors at the Autoimmunity Congress of 2012, which ordinarily permits only speakers who are doctors or scientists.

The examples of research into Helminth Therapy listed below, strongly suggest that within a decade, these parasitic worms, or drugs developed from them, could become potent treatments for patients with autoimmune conditions whose symptoms have not responded well to conventional medicine. It is most probable that helminth therapy would be superior to the current alternatives, and result in fewer side-effects.

University of Iowa immunologist David Elliott, who has studied helminths for more than a decade, is just one researcher who is optimistic about the future of this medical research:

> Our bodies, especially our immune systems, have evolved to expect input from these creatures. Without this feedback, the immune system can get badly off track....I can give a mouse multiple sclerosis, rheumatoid arthritis or colitis, and when I give it worms, the disease goes away. Can we do that in humans too? I don't see why not.

In 2005, Elliott and Dr Joel Weinstock, Chief of Gastroenterology and Hepatology at Tufts Medical Center in Boston, published statistics on two preliminary trials in humans. In one, involving 54 ulcerative colitis patients, 43% of those given pig whipworm eggs improved, compared with only 17% who received placebos. In a second trial 29 patients with Crohn's disease took whipworm eggs every 3 weeks. By the end of 24 weeks, 79% had reduced disease activity and a majority of these patients had gone into remission.

These results inspired researchers and biomedical companies around the world to investigate Helminth's potential for treating other conditions. Ultimately, the final aim of this research is to identify the particular molecules that allow these parasitic worms to benevolently control the immune system responses. If this is achieved, these molecules – or analogues of them – will be synthesized into medicines. *"By understanding what the worms do, we may be able to develop magic bullets,"* says Weinstock.

This approach would offer major advantages over using the worms themselves, because accurate and consistent dosing would be easy to control, and patients wouldn't be disgusted by the treatment. But this dream – if it ever becomes reality - will take a long time to materialize, and many researchers feel that a pharmaceutical product is unlikely, since helminths are exceptionally complex and use multiple mechanisms to achieve their objectives. *"It's hard to recreate complex biological interactions. These organisms are their own living drug-delivery systems. They have so many effects on their hosts,"* says Professor Parker.

P'ng Loke, Ph.D. Associate Professor of the New York State University Department of Microbiology (parasitology) documented the case of a Californian man he met in 2007, who had successfully treated his inflammatory bowel disease by self-medicating with parasitic worm eggs. He analysed the man's medical records prior to 2007 and personally tracked the man's health from 2007 onwards. The patient, who preferred to remain anonymous, was in his mid-30s when he was diagnosed with severe ulcerative colitis in 2003. He did not respond to steroid treatments, and his doctors eventually told him that surgery to remove his colon or immune system-suppressing therapy were his only hope.

He declined both options and instead, in 2004, he ingested 500 pig whipworm eggs, which he obtained from a parasitologist in Thailand. Three months later, he ingested another 1,000 eggs. By mid-2005, he was virtually symptom free and required no medical treatment, except for occasional anti-inflammatory drugs to suppress flare-ups. In 2008, when the number of whipworm eggs in the man's stool began to dwindle, the symptoms of colitis returned. The man infected himself with another 2,000 whipworm eggs and, a few months later, once again his symptoms almost vanished.

Repeated colonoscopies revealed that wherever worms colonized his colon, the open sores and inflammation, typical of colitis, disappeared or were considerably alleviated. In a paper published in *Science Translational Medicine*, Loke and his colleagues suggest that the whipworms are indeed effective in treating colitis. More importantly, Loke showed through tissue analysis that the parasites may work by stimulating mucus production in the gut. Colitis, which is associated with decreased mucus production, is thought to occur when the immune system attacks benign bacteria living in the intestines. The extra mucus triggered by the parasites may help calm the immune system, thereby preventing it from attacking the gut's harmless microorganisms.

More recent research results were published in 2011 by John Fleming, a neurologist at the University of Wisconsin, who pioneered the first MS-related clinical trial in the U.S. using TSO (pig whipworms). Five newly diagnosed MS patients drank TSO every two weeks for three months. Patients who took part said the liquid was salty but didn't taste or smell unpleasant. *"It was like drinking a shot of salty water—you didn't notice the worms. It wasn't like there was anything chunky in it,"* explains Jim, 40, the first patient recruited for Dr Fleming's safety study, who asked not to have his surname published.

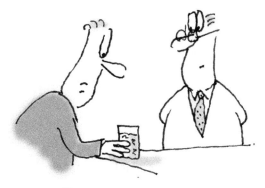

Am I allowed a whisky chaser?

Throughout the study, Fleming monitored new and old lesions (spots of nerve damage) in the brain and spinal cord, using MRI scans. Fleming found that lesions fell more than three-fold by the end of the study. When patients stopped drinking TSO, their lesions jumped back up to their original levels.

There has however, also occasionally been some bad news regarding Helminth Therapy studies. In October 2013, Coronado Biosciences of Burlington saw its stock tumble 67% after announcing the failure of its phase 2 clinical trial for the treatment of Crohn's disease. In their study, half of the 250 volunteers swallowed a drink containing 7,500 pig whipworm eggs every 2 weeks for 12 weeks. The other half drank a placebo, but for some inexplicable reason this particular trial did not meet its stated primary goal of significantly improving a measure of Crohn's disease severity, or a secondary goal of achieving remission.

Perhaps the most inspiring evidence for the potential efficacy of Helminth therapy is anecdotal, as can be seen from the following examples which relate amazing recoveries in the case of three individuals. The first suffering from chronic allergies, the second from Crohns disease and the third from severe autism:

Crohns Disease

In 2010, a Financial Analyst in New York, Herbert Smith, purchased pig and human whipworms and hookworms from Autoimmune Therapies and from Worm Therapy, via trips to Mexico and online mail-orders from Jasper. In 1996, Smith was diagnosed with Crohn's disease and subsequently had a foot of his intestines surgically removed before being inspired to try Helminth Therapy after reading about research conducted by Weinstock. He claims the hookworms triggered a complete remission and that he still remains free of Crohn's symptoms and can eat anything he wants, even high-fibre vegetables, without fear of triggering horrific symptoms. *"I'm living an entirely normal life,"* he says. *"This therapy could help people who don't have any other treatment options,"* Smith says.

- Readers can contact him via the following link to his Facebook page: http://www.facebook.com/Helminthic.Therapy

Chronic Allergies

A muscular, mid-forties, 200-pound blacksmith from Massachusetts, nicknamed Tom "Bear", used to suffer from hundreds of allergies. Potential allergens such as seafood, insect bites, pollen, and animal dander - substances that should have been perceived by his body as harmless or even beneficial - were all registered as life threatening and kept his immune system on high alert.

"As a kid I couldn't even eat green beans, I was deathly allergic to peanut butter. I couldn't touch my dog or my face would swell up. And if an insect bit me, the spot would stay swollen for 2 or 3 months." By

the time he reached adulthood, his condition had worsened and he frequently experienced suffocating asthma attacks.

A long-time friend of his who works as a technician at a university medical lab, came up with a cure: *"I knew that Bear's allergy to nuts in particular could kill him if he accidentally consumed them in processed foods and I knew I couldn't live with myself if he died and I could have stopped it"*, says the lab tech, who wishes to remain anonymous.

The friend's proposed remedy: intentional infection with eight tape-worm larvae he had harvested in the lab from a beetle and then washed, disinfected, and placed in a drinkable saline solution. The tapeworm used, though not specified, should have been rat tapeworms, since pig tapeworms are potentially lethal and beef tapeworms can also cause serious health issues. Bear drank this solution, and began to notice changes in his health between the second and third month.

"Nothing had been happening," Bear says, *"but the next thing I knew, I wasn't allergic to my dog anymore. I could put my face in his fur and my eyes didn't itch. I couldn't believe it—I didn't start sneezing. I had no allergic reaction at all."* For the first time in his life he could eat sushi, dunking raw seafood in soy sauce - a food combination which had been taboo and which now became his favourite meal. One late summer night, after eating half a bag of potato chips, he discovered that they had been fried in peanut oil—a likely death sentence before worm infection.

Severe Autism

Another amazing piece of anecdotal evidence - which has also been fully verified – concerns a boy with autism. In 2005 the Johnson family was at breaking point; Lawrence, the family's 13-year-old son, had been diagnosed with aggressive autism when two and a half years old and his parents had valiantly coped with his illness for the ensuing decade. Lawrence was given 1,000 pig whipworm (TSO) eggs every 2 weeks for 5 months, but there were no positive results until the dose was raised to 2,500 eggs every 2 weeks. Within 10 weeks of the higher-dose treatment, this autistic boy stopped smashing his head against the wall and no longer experienced fits during which he would gouge at his eyes.

The paralysis and frustration that held him and his family prisoners in their own home lifted, and the freak-outs ceased. *"It wasn't gradations. It just went away. All these behaviours just disappeared"*, remembers his father, Stewart, who had always kept meticulous notes on Lawrence's disorder. Lawrence's doctor, Eric Hollander, was stunned and asked Stewart to present the findings to his colleagues at the Seaver Autism Center at its annual conference in 2007. Stewart recalls; *"They were very impressed"* - so impressed that they used the case of Lawrence Johnson as the basis to apply for a more formal clinical trial testing of TSO in other autistic patients with severely disruptive and aggressive behaviours.

Lawrence Johnson, now 25 years old, continues to respond positively to treatment with TSO eggs. Because the parasites are regularly flushed from his system, he takes a dose of TSO as his father sees the need, which is roughly every 2 weeks. Though this costs Stewart and his family about €600 a month, he says the treatment has changed their lives and this is well worth the price; *"There're no words to describe it. It's like giving me my son back,"* he continues; *"or in many ways, like giving me a son that I didn't ever have."*

Since witnessing the positive effects of TSO on Lawrence's worst behaviours, Stewart has launched a website: www.autismtso.com which shares his family's experience and informs other parents of the progress of current research, such as the clinical trial at the Seaver Center. He has also written a chapter about his experience with TSO treatment in the recently published *'Textbook of Autism Spectrum Disorders'*.

- Readers interested in the potential for using helminths to treat autism can listen to three lectures on the subject which Stewart presented to the 'Mount Sinai Autism Conference' in October 2007. https://www.youtube.com/watch?v=r_R_sHV8H9o; https://www.youtube.com/watch?v=4_O7Dp2Gud4; https://www.youtube.com/watch?v=oFnJZsFovuM.

Readers who wish to use helminth therapy should note that, although there are currently a number of retailers who supply live worms to customers, some seem highly questionable. Therefore, if forced, I would only be willing to recommend the following company:

- Biome Restoration https://biomerestoration.com/products

Biome Restoration was founded by Judy Chinitz and Marc Dellerba, who cooperated with the Medicines and Healthcare Products Regulatory Agency and consequently they are permitted to sell the organisms as non-pharmaceutical products. More importantly, Dellerba has a PhD in Chemistry and oversees a rigorous manufacturing process.

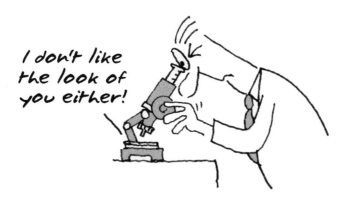

Chinitz and Dellerba began their helminth supply company in the UK three years ago, and today have more than 1,200 regular customers. They ship all over the world, microscopic larvae which grow into worms after being swallowed. Legally, this is somewhat of a grey area, since theoretically it is breaching the law: many health regulatory agencies, including those in the UK and US, deem most helminths to be pathogens that should not be transported.

The following is a list of other helminth producers:

- Jasper Lawrence's company - www.autoimmunetherapies.com

- Biomonde - www.biomonde-asia.com/english/home/home.html

- Coronado Biosciences - www.coronadobiosciences.com

- Ovamed GmbH - www.ovamed.org/

- WormTherapy - www.wormtherapy.com

Some people are now taking the DIY route and are raising helminths themselves. William Parker estimates that circa 7,000 people worldwide have used worms as a medicine over the past few years, and based on the evidence that he and other researchers have gathered from hundreds of users, he says that helminth therapy; *"has a really good benefit-to-risk ratio, especially for serious auto-immune diseases such as multiple sclerosis and inflammatory bowel disorder."*

There are also online communities where helminth enthusiasts can discuss the best worm-raising regimens and most effective dosing strategies. I recommend that readers interested in this area begin their journey of exploration with the following FAQ sheet can be found on Jasper Lawrence's website:

• https://autoimmunetherapies.com/ documents/FAQ.pdf.

The following YouTube videos featuring Jasper Lawrence and Garin Aglietti may be of interest to some readers:

• https://www.youtube.com/user/jascallaw

A discussion on helminth therapy by Asphelia Pharmaceuticals can be found here:

• https://www.youtube.com/watch?v=uzEI5wKO13Y)

Finally, I would like to emphasise that although helminth therapy is available at some private clinics in Europe and Tijuana in Mexico, readers should beware of attending these establishments as this treatment has not yet been approved in the US or Europe. In addition, Professor Weinstock cautions that; *"People shouldn't be buying these things over the internet as there are definite dangers involved due to taking wrong doses or purchasing dangerous or contaminated worms"*.

Having said this however, for the sake of curious readers, a man with Crohn's disease who ignored Professor Weinstock's advice and infected himself with worms can be viewed at

• https://www.youtube.com/watch?v=_fwV-btDwww

In case this video inspires someone to opt for helminthic self-infestation without any medical supervision, here is the 'antidote' that should serve to make them change their mind. The following two videos reveal the potential negative side-effects of worm infestation and should convince anyone considering this treatment to adhere to Professor Weinstock's aforementioned advice regarding medical supervision:

The dark side of a hookworm infestation:

- https://www.youtube.com/watch?v=g5QWhMKu-vF8&list=PLeMsTfnnZppxs-shl%20_wtfcorfmg7vOpC0

The dark side of a tapeworm infection:

- https://www.youtube.com/watch?v=m9F1EhfvYpA#password

Some interesting articles on helminth therapy available on-line:

- Scientific Studies of Helminthic Therapy: http://www.foodsmatter.com/natural_medicine_comp_therapies/helminthic_therapy/articles/helminthic-therapy-reading-list-05-12.pdf

- New York Times article published in July 2008: http://www.nytimes.com/2008/07/01/health/research/01prof.html?_r=0

- Helminthic therapy article on NHS online news site in 2009: http://www.nhs.uk/news/2009/01January/Pages/WormsImmuneSystem.aspx

- The Guardian – article on Jasper Lawrence's story published in May 2010: http://www.theguardian.com/lifeandstyle/2010/may/23/parasitic-hookworm- jasper-lawrence-tim-adams

- Scientific American - article on helminth therapy published in December 2010: http://www.scientificamerican.com/article/helminthic-therapy-mucus/

- The Scientist – article on helminth therapy and autism published in February 2011:

http://www.the-scientist.com/?articles.view/articleNo/29485/
title/Opening-a-Can-of-Worms/

- Wall Street Journal – article on helminth therapy published in June 2011:
  http://www.wsj.com/articles/SB10001424052702304314404576
  413303666083390

- New Scientist – article on helminth therapy published in August 2011:
  https://www.newscientist.com/article/mg21128243-500-let-them-eat-worms/

- Men's Health Magazine –anecdotal information published in November 2012:
  http://www.menshealth.com/health/immune-system-worms

- science Daily – article published in August 2014:
  https://www.sciencedaily.com/releases/2014/08/140811125126.htm

- The Guardian – article published in February 2016:
  http://www.theguardian.com/lifeandstyle/2016/feb/08/why-a-diet-of-worms-could-be-good-for-you

CHAPTER SIX

CUTTING EDGE APITHERAPY

Apitherapy (from the Latin word for bee, "*apis*") which uses bee venom as well as pollen, honey, and other hive products to prevent or treat illness and injuries, may be as old as human medicine itself. Early hunter-gatherers drew images on rocks depicting the honeybee as a source of medical treatment, and references to bee-stings as an effective cure for arthritis and joint pains can be found in medical texts. These are thousands of years' old, dating back to the three great ancient civilizations of Egypt, Greece, and China who were known for their evolved healthcare systems.

Apitherapy has cured my arthritis

How much did they sting you for that?

The beneficial effect of bee stings on swollen joints can be attributed to mellitin, an anti-inflammatory agent, known to be a hundred times stronger than cortisone. Since this therapeutic system dates back thousands of years, and we know that in pseudoscience circles, age is a perfectly valid substitute for "evidence that it actually works", and given the fact that bee venom is 100% natural - another substitute for effectiveness - this perhaps explains in part its steadily increasing popularity and the exaggerated claims regarding apitherapy's healing potential.

Indeed, there are increasing numbers of 'complimentary alternative medicine', acupuncturists, homeopaths, and even doctors, who currently advocate it for the treatment of various autoimmune diseases including rheumatoid arthritis, osteoarthritis, shingles, tendonitis, gout, carpal tunnel syndrome, Lou Gehrig's disease, fibromyalgia, painful scars and burns, multiple sclerosis (MS), and Lyme disease.

Doctors of traditional Chinese medicine have relied on bee sting therapy for centuries. "Wang Menglin, a 'bee acupuncturist' who works in a Beijing clinic in China, says he has *treated patients with dozens of diseases, from arthritis to cancer, all with positive results.*" Indeed Apitherapy is more popular in China than anywhere else in the world; thousands of practitioners claim almost unbelievable results from their treatments, which not only employ bee venom but also countless other bee-products. However, perhaps this exaggerated enthusiasm for Apitherapy has been influenced by the fact that these 'medical' therapists receive support and funding from the Chinese government who sell Chinese Apitherapy products worldwide, comprising $84 billion USD in goods.

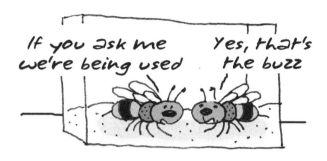

According to the National Bureau of Statistics, Apitherapy merchandise makes up more than 31 percent of the entire country's medicine output. *"Globally, it's a huge system of medicine, especially in Asia, Europe, the Middle East, and South America, where even many MDs sting their patients,"* says Frederique Keller, LAc, apitherapist, acupuncturist, and president of the American Apitherapy Society (AAS), headquartered in Centerport, New York.

In 2004, South Korean researchers published a study, *"Anti-arthritic Effect of Bee Venom,"* in which they gave rats with advanced rheumatoid arthritis low doses of bee venom. Apparently, the venom dramatically reduced tissue swelling and osteophyte formation on affected paws, showing a correlation between the anti-inflammatory properties and anti-arthritis effects of bee venom.

And yet strangely, there is *zero* scientific evidence in the West to confirm that Apitherapy is a useful treatment option for any of the aforementioned diseases. Furthermore, the treatment can produce rare but dangerous side effects, including inflammation of the central nervous system. Although less than 1 percent of the population is allergic to bee venom, in those people a sting can cause anaphylactic shock and even death, so one of the first rules for anyone using apitherapy is to have an EpiPen (containing epinephrine) nearby and to know how to use it at the first signs of throat constriction or difficulty in breathing. Additionally, in rare cases, bee venom can also trigger optic neuritis which happens to be common in people with MS and which can lead to significant visual impairment.

The popularity of Apitherapy in the United States can largely be attributed to Charles Mraz, nicknamed "The Bee Man," a beekeeper from New York who first advocated bee venom therapy in the 1930s after using it effectively to treat his own arthritis. He was inspired by Bodeg Beck, a Hungarian who moved to America after World War I, and brought apitherapy to the United States. Mraz asserted that the anti-inflammatory response mounted against the bee sting serves to reduce other inflammatory processes throughout the body, and he treated people with bee stings for arthritis pain for over sixty years.

Charles was also a founding member of the American Apitherapy Society, authoring the book *Health and The Honey Bee* in 1994, which recounted his experiences with BVT, where in a typical treatment session, 20-40 bees are used. The bee is grasped with tweezers and placed on a specific body part. After the sting, the stinger is allowed to remain for 10 to 15 minutes. To reduce pain, ice is sometimes used to numb the area before and after the sting. The location of the sting definitely matters - most apitherapy users sting where the pain occurs and along the spine (to stimulate bloodflow and neurotransmitters).

Practitioners are discovering that stinging at acupuncture points gives your body an added boost by opening qi channels, says Frederique Keller. The number of stings you get, and how often you get them, varies with each person. Someone with tennis elbow, for example, might need just two stings a week for three weeks, while someone with Lyme disease, or MS, might need several sessions a week for many months, comprising of 10 or more stings at each session.

The growing popularity of Bee-sting Therapy in the Western world, in spite of the absence of scientific support is mainly due to anecdotal 'evidence', like the story of 59 year old Kathleen Miller of Albuquerque. In order to treat her arthritic, severely damaged knee, she turned to bee venom, because she had read stories about its alleged pain-relieving and anti-inflammatory properties. Previously a world-class marathon runner in the 1980's, she placed fifth at the 1980 Boston Marathon, but her high impact hobby, wore out her right knee, and in 1990, she tore her cartilage while rock climbing. She chose surgery, and was running a month later, but a year after this, after tearing the cartilage a second time, on this occasion, while swimming, she again underwent surgery but this time her knee *"stayed in a postoperative condition: incredibly red, hot, swollen, and painful,"* and for the next four years she lived on a maximum dosage of ibuprofen and other nonsteroidal anti-inflammatory drugs which offered only very limited relief.

At the age of 47, after enduring more surgery, then acupuncture, as well as various other treatments, she applied, in desperation, for knee replacement surgery. But in spring 1996 after hearing about a farmer whose rheumatoid arthritis was cured when he put on his pyjamas and was stung by a bee which had been hiding in the trouser leg, she began researching apitherapy, and subsequently, in the same year ordered a "bee box", which contained dozens of bees including candy paste for the bees to eat.

She stung herself, and for the following two days her knee ballooned up, severely swollen, and fiery red. Apparently, this was an ideal physical reaction to the treatment as it meant her immune system was responding in the required manner, whereas sometimes multiple stings are needed to stimulate a sufficient immune response to the procedure. On the third day the swelling subsided, and her knee was one-third smaller than it had been in four years. *"For the first time, the 'heat' in the knee was gone, too,"* she says. So she continued stinging herself three times a week. A couple of months later, she claimed that she could once again swim, lift weights, take long walks and handle the gardening. Fifteen months after this, she reduced her treatment to a single 'maintenance sting' every few months, which was sufficient in maintaining her knee health.

The story of Pat Wagner is perhaps even more impressive than Kathleen's: Pat treats herself for multiple sclerosis (MS) by allowing bees to sting her, and she has come to be known as "The Bee Woman" by advocating bee venom therapy after claiming to have effectively treated her own illness.

She calls this bee-venom therapy (BVT) and genuinely believes it has saved her from MS. She was diagnosed at Georgetown University Hospital in the spring of 1970 with relapsing/remitting multiple sclerosis and received numerous medications that ultimately failed to help. This was because her MS worsened over the years until the spring of 1992 when she failed to respond to two courses of high-dose Prednisone and became wheelchair bound, suffering from bladder incontinence which was not helped by bladder surgery.

Then, on March 24, 1992, she received her first intentional sting from a honeybee. After just two days, there was a noticeable increase in energy evidenced by her ability to remain awake for a significantly longer time in the daytime. More importantly, she regained the MS-related lost hearing in the right ear and within two weeks of the receiving the stings, no longer required her wheelchair.

Thanks to stories like this, there are up to 10,000 people with MS currently undergoing this same type of treatment, administering BVT to themselves or others, often with the assistance of unlicensed practitioners, since the treatment cannot legally be prescribed by a doctor as a medical treatment.

If indeed bee venom *has* genuinely helped some MS sufferers, its therapeutic effects may be due to the presence of the chemical Apamin, a component of bee venom which has been shown to inhibit the potassium channel, the same part of the nerve cell inhibited by the experimental drug 4-aminopyridine, that has also shown promising results for MS-associated fatigue, leg weakness, and walking difficulty. However, in spite of the various isolated reports of people with MS experiencing a significant reduction in symptoms following bee venom therapy, as in the case of Pat Wagner, larger studies do not seem to indicate any significant benefits whatsoever from this treatment.

In the Netherlands in 2004, the results of a high-quality clinical study using extensive clinical and MRI measures to investigate the efficacy of bee venom therapy on MS claimed zero benefits to MS sufferers observed in terms of MRI measurements, MS attacks, progression of disability, fatigue, or quality of life.

However, there is one piece of research within the field of Apitherapy, which may well have a future. A potential cancer treatment has recently been developed, using a synthetic version of the active ingredient of bee venom, Mellitin (that doesn't trigger the kind of allergic reactions to bee stings that other components of bee venom do), and the results of this treatment so far seem promising.

Melittin's anti-tumour potential has been known for years, but it hasn't been used as a drug because it also attacks healthy cells, including vital red blood cells. However one group of researchers, using 'nanotechnology', have found a way to surmount this problem. The study, which was funded by the National Institutes of Health, and the American Heart Association, was carried out by scientists from Washington University School of Medicine, USA. The objective of the research was to examine the effects of Mellitin, on cancer cells.

Mellitin kills both healthy and diseased cells in mammals by attaching itself to the surface of cells and ripping holes in the surrounding membrane as well as in the important structures within the cells. *"In high enough concentration it can destroy any cell it comes into contact with,"* said Professor Paul Schlesinger, a cell biologist at Washington University.

Most cancer treatments target DNA, but cancer cells are frequently able to adapt and develop resistance to DNA damage. It is much harder for cells to defend against damage to the membrane, and it is this fact which potentially makes Mellitin an especially attractive cancer treatment, assuming clinical trials conclude that it *is* a viable option.

The researchers discovered a method for incorporating Mellitin into tiny molecules, "nanoparticles" which can be programmed to attack and destroy *only* cancer cells, while leaving healthy non-cancerous cells intact. The carrier particles, nicknamed "nanobees", attack newly forming cancers by targeting the leaky blood vessels surrounding them, which feed the cancerous tumours. *"The nanobees 'fly in', land on the surface of cells and deposit their poisonous cargo,"* said Professor Samuel Wickline, the specialist in nanomedicine who led the research at Washington University.

The nanobees, which are spherical, about six millionths of an inch in diameter, and made of perfluorocarbon, an inert non-toxic compound used in artificial blood, are rapidly cleared from the body once they have completed their task; because after depositing the Mellitin, they dissolve and are evaporated in the lungs.

The treatment was tested on three types of tumour in live mice: mouse melanoma skin cancers, precancerous lesions caused by human papillomavirus, (which can cause cervical cancer in humans), and a form of human breast cancer transplanted into the mice.

The results of the study, published in 2009 in *The Journal of Clinical Investigation*, a peer-reviewed journal, indicated that mice injected with Mellitin-containing nanoparticles over 18 days (one injection every 3 days) showed no evidence of rupture of healthy blood cells, no physiological signs of adverse effects and no evidence of damage to the liver, lungs, kidney and heart. In the mice that had been transplanted with human breast cancer cells, there was a 25% reduction in tumour size as compared with control injections (salt water). The size of mouse melanoma tumours decreased by approximately 88% in comparison to the untreated mice; the treatment also proved effective in targeting and reducing the size of pre-cancerous cells.

The researchers concluded from these results, that synthetic nanoparticles can be used successfully to deliver Mellitin, which kills both established tumours and pre-cancerous lesions. Additionally, these "nanobees" could eventually replace conventional therapy for certain types of cancer because the treatment would have fewer side-effects than chemotherapy.

More recently, in February 2013, it was reported that nanoparticles carrying Mellitin were also effective in destroying HIV by eroding the double-layer viral envelope surrounding the virus. Possible applications include a vaginal gel that would target HIV intrusion prior to infection, as well as an intravenous treatment that would be applicable in the case of already-existing HIV infections.

According to the NHS, however, all this research is still at a very early stage and its effects have only been tested over a short period of time and limited to mice. A great deal more research yielding positive results with other 'test animals' will be required before it could be deemed potentially safe for testing in humans.

To end on a lighter note, apparently Gwyneth Paltrow uses bee-sting therapy as a beauty treatment. Taking into account the scarcity of healthy bees and the fact that stinging is potentially a death sentence for them, some might condemn those who opt for this beauty treatment as behaving in an extremely selfish fashion, especially given the incredibly superficial reason for sacrificing such a benevolent creature. In addition, the manner of death worsens the situation, since the barb in a bee's stinger rips out its abdomen as it flies away, causing massive internal trauma to the bee that is followed by a painful death.

However, since Gwyneth is a supporter of vegetarianism, veganism and the animal rights organization Peta, she uses another far less unpleasant method for accessing bee-venom, in the form of a bee-venom 'facial', which involves 'milking' bees in a way which does *not* kill or significantly harm them.

Unlike the bee-sting treatment, the facial blends the venom with UMF 18+ Manuka Honey, applying it like a regular face mask, after first using a tiny swab of the bee-venom behind the client's ear to ensure no allergic reaction. The venom is extracted using a small electrically charged metal plate placed inside the hive, which the bee finds threatening and attacks, but because the plate is hard, the venom is released without loss of the sting, so the bee survives to sting again, and the venom can be scraped off.

There is a light stinging effect from the venom face mask, which draws blood to the area and stimulates the production of collagen and elastin – natural components of the skin which have profoundly beneficial effects on skin quality, in contrast to synthetic versions of these same chemicals that form the ingredients of various expensive cosmetic creams that serve no useful purpose whatsoever.

Collagen (from the Greek *"kolla,"* meaning glue), consists of superfine protein fibres (fibrils) - gram for gram stronger than steel - which form a 'scaffold' that maintains the strength and structure of our skin. Likewise, the protein Elastin keeps the skin both tight and elastic, allowing it to resume its shape after stretching or contracting. Collagen and elastin production decline with age and exposure to UV light, and the loss of the skin's strong structural support and elasticity causes sagging of the skin, lines and wrinkles.

Bee-venom facials seem to be a favourite trend among celebrity figures such as Simon Cowell, Kylie Minogue and Victoria Beckham. Some even regard interacting with live bees as a type of meditation: Sara Mapelli is an energy therapist who dances while adorned with a swarm of bees and she told the National Geographic that the sensation is *"itchy, a little painful, and their little feet pinch my skin as they tightly grip on, while others climb over them. But it's all part of the experience, part of the meditation."*

CHAPTER SEVEN

BEER-SPA THERAPY

Alleged to be an authentic "medical" procedure, Beer Spas have existed for hundreds of years, though in this century it is the Czech's who have catalysed their re-emergence and popularity. Enthusiasts claim that they increase pulmonary circulation, lower blood pressure and revitalize the nervous system. The active beer yeast provides the skin with a wide range of vitamins B, proteins and saccharides, contributing to an overall softening and rejuvenation of the entire body. The sweating induced by the heat of the water eliminates toxins, cleansing the pores and regenerating hair and skin. The nutrient-rich bath is even supposed to speed up the healing process of open wounds and alleviate the symptoms of psoriasis and acne.

However, to achieve these considerable effects, it is essential that the bath is maintained at a constant temperature of 37 degrees Celsius. The ingredients must be natural, pure and correctly balanced and the water used in the spa has to be mineral water, not tap water.

The bathing experience takes place in specially designed tubs and the spa should be continuously bubbling to facilitate the dissolving of the barley, hops, beer yeast and dehydrated crushed herbs. These nutrient-rich ingredients penetrate the open skin pores to purify tired skin, and soften tense muscles.

Perhaps most important of all, bathing in the spa, combined simultaneously with the imbibing of the finest quality unpasteurized beer made from the purest of ingredients, triggers a powerful endorphin rush to create a most outstanding anti-stress treatment that re-establishes, at least for a while, a genuine sense of inner balance and harmony.

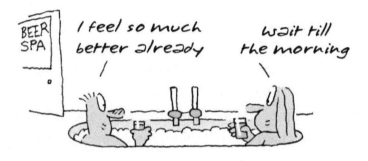

The session is complete after the client receives a massage culminating with a 30 minute 'deep-rest' period in the 'relaxation zone,' where the peaceful ambience is enhanced by dimmed lighting and soothing music. Here, clients rest quietly on a bed, covered by a sheet and a fleece quilt which encourages the skin to further absorb all the nutrients from the bath.

The entire procedure lasts one and a half hours and it should come as no surprise to learn that most customers leave the experience thoroughly rejuvenated with a feeling of calm and spiritual well-being, characterized by a gentle flow of positive thoughts and calm energy. It is said that to gain maximum health benefits from this trip, that bathers should refrain from showering afterwards for at least 12 hours which allows for a full assimilation of the enlivening ingredients.

It is recommended that for those with healthy immune systems it is sufficient to repeat the procedure just once a month to gain significant benefits, whereas individuals who are constantly stressed or who frequently feel unwell are invited to participate twice a week in order to improve their health and wellbeing.

Contra-indication: The Beer Spa is not appropriate for people with high blood pressure, or for those who have undergone recent heart surgery, and it is not allowed in the case of pregnant women from the third month of pregnancy or for children below the age of 15.

The sizes of the baths vary according to which beer spa one visits. The beer spas in the Czech Republic offer hot tubs suitable for one or two people, whereas at the *Schloss Starkenberger Beer Spa* in Austria, in the castle's 700-year-old cellar, the old fermentation rooms have been modified to allow for seven, 13 foot long, wide metal vats that are actually old fermenting tanks, repurposed to be safe to bathe in and these can easily take as many as ten clients.

However, beer lovers should note that although the "*Beer Spa Bernard*" in the centre of Prague as well as other beer spas in the Czech Republic allow you, whilst bathing, to pour yourself as many beers as you wish from the bath-side beer tap, the same rules do not apply in the *Austrian* beer spa, as the brewery has made it clear to the public that drinking while bathing is "*streng verboten*" (strictly forbidden).

Ragus, an Irishman whom the author interviewed, spent a week at the Beer Spa Bernard in the centre of Prague, and nicely sums up the sort of experience that visitors can expect. His surname has been omitted since he needs to remain anonymous owing to a serious drink problem that caused his employer to give him an ultimatum: teetotal....or redundant.

The author asked Ragus to encapsulate his experience in a short review, and this is what he wrote:

> The wonderful and wide-ranging health benefits of the Beer Spa in Prague have stood the test of time since the practice began in the middle Ages. The luxuriously warm, continuously bubbling, foaming caramel coloured, life-giving fluid you bathe in, and the deliciously cool amber nectar that infuses your entire being with joy as it slides smoothly down your throat, are brewed only from all-natural ingredients including the finest hops and purest of spring water, and after you have finished pouring from a personal tub-side tap, as much of the company's home-brewed Beer as takes your fancy, your sumptuous mind-body experience concludes with a sensuous 20-minute massage enhanced by a final relaxation session on a heated bed enveloped by the tantalizing aromas of freshly brewed beer. With your body being treating from inside and outside in this mind-blowing way, the yeast you can expect, is to leave the treatment wonderfully invigorated, feeling like a new man, no matter what ales you!

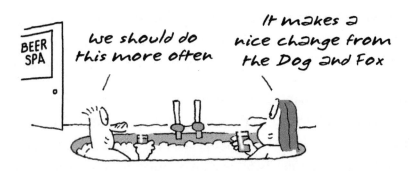

The treatments vary in price from spa to spa but are in the region of €100 per person for the full package including massage.

The following website lists and describes all six Beer Spas in the Czech Republic:

- http://travelaway.me/beer-spas/

The first and perhaps currently the *only* beer spa in the USA

- http://www.hopinthespa.com/

The Schloss Starkenberger beer spa in Austria

- http://www.starkenberger.at/das-bierbad-geschenk.html

Lightning Source UK Ltd.
Milton Keynes UK
UKHW050159020320
359580UK00018BA/372